# Da Yan
# Wild Goose Qigong

## The 2nd
## 64 Movements

大雁氣功
后六十四式

**Simon Blow**

☯

First published 2014
Copyright © 2014 Simon Blow

National Library of Australia
Cataloguing-in-Publication data:

Da Yan Wild Goose Qigong – The 2nd 64 Movements

ISBN: 978-0-9873417-2-3

Published by:
Genuine Wisdom Centre
PO Box 446
Summer Hill NSW 2130
Australia
(www.genuinewisdomcentre.com)

Editing:
www.essencewriting.com.au
www.mediawords.com.au


Cover design and layout:
Determind Design (www.determind.com.au)

Diagrams:
John Bennetts (johnbennettsmusic.com)

**Disclaimer**
The intention of this book is to present information and practices that have been used throughout China for many years. The information offered is according to the author's best knowledge and is to be used by the reader at his or her own discretion and liability. Readers should obtain professional advice where appropriate regarding their health and health practices. The author disclaims all responsibility and liability to any person, arising directly or indirectly from taking or not taking action based upon the information in this publication.

This book is dedicated to

To Grand Master Chen Chuan Gang and Madam Chen for welcoming me into the Da Yan family and giving me guidance on this path.

# Contents

Acknowledgements                                             X

About the author                                             XI

Romanisation of Chinese words                                XII

How to use this book                                         XIII

Chapter 1: Introduction                                      1

Chapter 2: Wu Wei – The Essence of Da Yan Qigong             5

Chapter 3: A Continuing Journey                              11

Chapter 4: The Art of Practice                               23

Chapter 5: Qigong Preparation Movements                      33

Chapter 6: The 2nd 64 Movements                              57

Chapter 7: Gathering the Qi and Rubbing the Face             169

Chapter 8: Meridian Charts                                   175

Chapter 9: Stories to Inspire                                197

Book/DVDs and CDs by Simon Blow                              204

Other Services and Products                                  212

Bibliography                                                 213

**Plum Blossoms**, Grand Master Tang Cheng Qing, Qing Cheng Shan
Green City Mountain, Sichuan Province, China September 2013

# Acknowledgements

There are many people I would like to thank for helping me to compile and develop this book.

Since I started teaching full-time in 1992, I have been teaching many classes each week for the general public and within therapeutic communities. I have had the great opportunity to meet many people on their own healing journey and I have been inspired by their stories. I get many ideas and positive feedback from all the people I meet and from those who have generously shared their own experiences in this book. I'm not sure if we have original ideas or if, when the heart opens and the Qi flows, we are simply all one. Again, thank you.

I would like to thank all who have attended my classes, workshops and residential retreats over the years. Also to those who have travelled with me to China. Without all your help and support I would not have been able to continue on this path.

My great appreciation to Grand Master Chen Chuan Gang and Madam Chen for sharing their wisdom and insight with me and for accepting me into the Da Yan Wild Goose family. I feel very honoured that they have given me the opportunity to write these books and document their family legacy so all can benefit. As we have discussed many times; it's all meant to be, it's destiny. A special thank you to Zhang Jing, my Daoist brother and business partner. You have educated me and enriched my life with your friendship and guidance, allowing me to gain a deeper understanding of Chinese culture. Your expert translations and assistance in introducing me to many esteemed masters has allowed me to grow and understand and share the complexities of this ancient healing art.

I would like to thank Lynn Guilhaus and Elizabeth Bond for proofreading and editing and for bringing this project to life. Thank you John Bennetts for the original photos and drawing adaptations; every diagram is a work of art. Master Zhang Cheng Cheng for the original Chinese writing and Grand Master Tang Cheng Qing for the beautiful paintings. Thank you to Mamun Khan and all his team from Determind Design for the layout and design.

We refer to Qigong as an art form. It is a process of refining our internal energy to harmonise with the external energy or environment. It's our own observation of our relationship with everything around us. We are influenced by everything around us; we are one with everything.

# About the Author: Simon Blow

A near fatal accident at the age of nineteen led Simon to investigate various methods of healing and rejuvenation, a path he has been following ever since. Simon is a Sydney-based (Australia) master teacher (Laoshi) of the ancient Chinese art of longevity and has been leading regular classes for beginning and continuing students since 1990.

Having travelled the world to learn and explore this ancient art, Simon has received extensive training and certification from many respected sources: Traditional lineage Grand Masters, Traditional Chinese Medical hospitals and Daoist monasteries in China, Buddhist monasteries in Australia, and Hindu ashrams in India. He has been given authority to share these techniques through his teachings and publications.

Simon has received extensive personal training in the Da Yan Wild Goose Qigong from the 28th generation lineage holder Grand Master, Chen Chuan Gang, and is an initinated student and 29th generation of this ancient healing art.

He received World Health Organisation certification in medical Qigong clinical practice from the Xiyuan Hospital in Beijing and is a Standing Council Member of the World Academic Society of Medical Qigong in Beijing. He has also been initiated into Dragon Gate Daoism and given the name of Xin Si, meaning 'genuine wisdom'.

Simon has spent quality time on many occasions at the Ramana Ashram in Southern India under the sacred mountain of Arunachala, following the self-realisation practices of Sri Ramana Maharishi.

His dedication, compassion and wisdom also make Simon a sought-after keynote speaker, workshop and retreat facilitator. By demand he has created a series of Book/DVD sets and guided meditation CDs. He also helped produce CDs for the Sunnatram Forest Monastery, the YWCA Encore program and a series of Meditation CDs for children and teenagers.

China holds a special place in Simon's heart. He has had the great fortune to travel to China on many occasions to study Qigong, attend international conferences, tour the sacred mountains and experience the rich culture of the Chinese people. Since 1999 he has been leading unique study tours to China so he could take people to the source and give them the opportunity to experience first-hand this ancient healing practice.

# Romanisation of Chinese words

The Genuine Wisdom Centre uses the Pinyin romanisation system of Chinese to English. Pinyin is a name for the system used to transliterate Chinese words into the Roman alphabet. The use of Pinyin was first adopted in the 1950s by the Chinese government, and it became official in 1979 when it was endorsed by the People's Republic of China.

Pinyin is now standard in the People's Republic of China and in several world organisations, including the United Nations. Pinyin replaces the Wade-Giles and Yale systems.

Some common conversions:

| Pinyin | Also spelled as | Pronunciation |
| --- | --- | --- |
| Qi | Chi | Chee |
| Qigong | Chi Kung | Chee Kung |
| Tai Ji | Tai Chi | Tai Jee |
| Taijiquan | Tai Chi Chuan | Tai Jee Chuen |
| Gongfu | Kung Fu | Gong Foo |
| Dao | Tao | Dao |
| Daoism | Taoism | Daoism |
| Dao De Jing | Tao Teh Ching | Dao Teh Ching |

## The use of Chinese characters in this publication

Chinese writing has been a developing medium for thousands of years and is the oldest continuously used system of writing in the world. It's the foundation of many of the other Asian styles of writing, originating from simple pictures to complex brush strokes with many thousands of individual characters. Since the 1950s, traditional characters which numbered to the tens of thousands have been simplified to four or five thousand. Even though there are many different dialects spoken in China, including Mandarin and Cantonese, the characters remain the same and their written technique and meaning are taught in all schools across China. The computerised font used for Chinese characters which are used today and in this publication are simplified Chinese and some of the deeper meaning or essence from the ancient times has been lost in the translation from traditional to simplified characters.

A good example is the word 'Qi' as written in Pinyin or sometimes written as 'Chi', which is used to describe the energy of life or life-force energy.

氣 The traditional character for Qi shows a picture of a pot being heated on a fire or cooking of rice with steam smouldering from the top as a result of the cooking or the refining process of cultivating the internal energy.

气 The simplified character for Qi only shows the steam rising and is sometimes translated as air or breath, losing the deeper understanding of cultivation or refinement.

## How to use this book

Da Yan Wild Goose Qigong is a very complex dynamic set of exercises. The book gives detailed instructions on how to perform the movements and provides additional theory and history to complement the practices. To view videos showing the shape of the movements
please visit out YouTube channel
**www.youtube.com/simonblowqigong**

It's important to learn from an experienced qualified teacher and to practise reguarly to master the movements yourself. Attending regular classes provides consistent practice and refinement and the energy of the group nurtures and supports everyone. It's important not to stray too far from the flock.

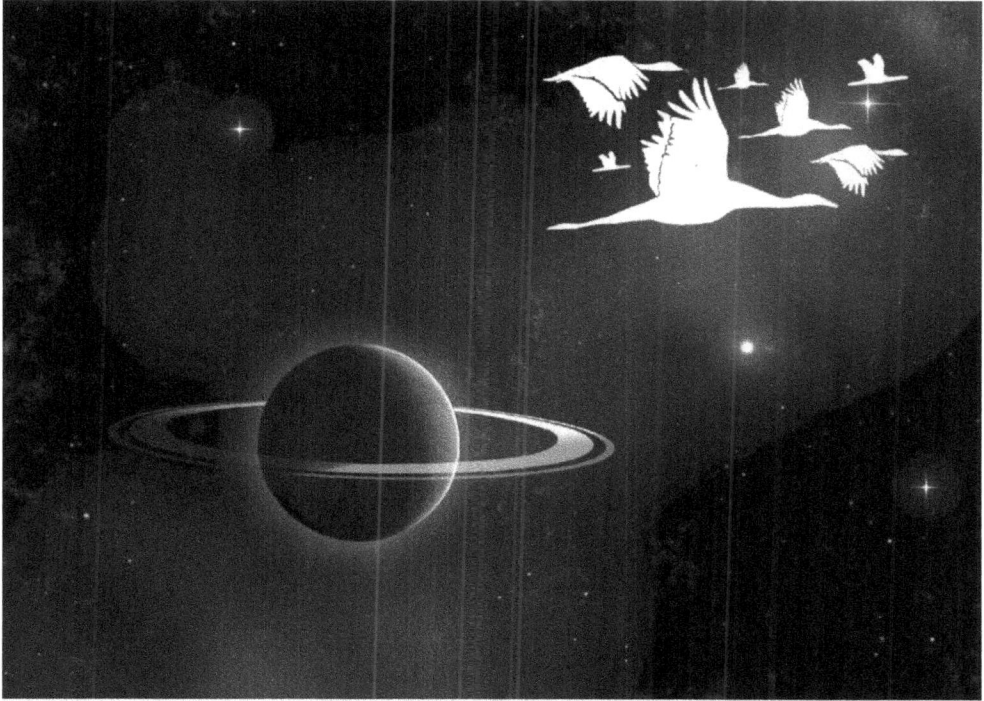

# Chapter 1
# Introduction

Da Yan - Wild Goose Qigong
The 2nd 64 movements

# Introduction

The Da Yan Wild Goose Qigong is one of the great treasures of the Chinese healing arts. It has been cultivated and nurtured for over a thousand years. The Da Yan or wild goose is a high energy bird which flies thousands of kilometres from one side of the world to the other and over 10 000 meters high over the mountains. In many cultures it is considered a messenger between heaven and earth, taking us to the next life. The Da Yan is a symbol of love and peace; it takes us on a journey to rediscover the beauty of the world that we live in.

The 2nd 64 movement set of the Da Yan Wild Goose Qigong follows on from where the 1st 64 movement set finishes. They complement one another, with the prenatal (before heaven) harmonising with the postnatal (after heaven); the external Qi merging with the internal Qi, making us whole and allowing our consciousness to become naturally in harmony with the universe. It's only when we have mastered the movements, details and Qi flow of the 1st 64 movement set that we can start to study the 2nd 64 movement set and for the full benefits to be realised.

The repetitive practice of the 1st 64 movement set will purge the organ meridians or energy channels of the body and stimulate the small and large heavenly orbit. The orbits help to strengthen and increase the natural process of refining Jing (essence) into Qi (energy) and through the clarity of the mind the Qi transforms into Shen (spiritual energy). The 2nd 64 movement set bridges between intermediate and advanced practice; the twisting, stretching, bending and pressing movements produce stronger Qi fields and intensify the circulation of the eight extraordinary channels. We refine our spiritual energy by returning to nothingness, leading a virtuous life and allowing ourselves to merge with the divine or Dao.

There is no easy way. It's through the practical training and practice that we feel and understand the Qi. It has to be done thousands of times over a number of years to fully cleanse the body's energy system to allow this natural alchemic process to happen. We harmonise the external Yang energy by gathering heavenly Qi from the planets, moon, mountains and water and combine it with the internal Yin energy of our original Qi and the energy we receive through food and the air that we breathe. This harmonising of Yin and Yang forms life itself.

An ancient Chinese saying describing the heavenly orbit: 'If water and fire of the human body coordinate with each other, one will be thriving in spirit and adequate in Qi and no evil Qi dare attack us.'

The theory, philosophy and basic principles presented in the 1st 64 movement set book carry on to the 2nd 64 movement set and a good practical understanding is required before commencing the 2nd 64 movement set. The main principle is the practice; the movements help to stimulate and increase our Qi field and when this happens the theory will make more sense.

The first level of training focuses on learning the form, the shape of each posture and the sequence of movements. The second level of training focuses on learning all the details, which includes the major meridians' acupoints. The third level of training focuses on learning the Qi or energy flow. If the movement is not correct, clear and accurate, the details will not be correct and then the Qi flow will not be correct.

Daoist thought generally focuses on nature and our relationship with humanity and the cosmos. 'The Dao' is 'the way of life' or a method of living in harmony with the Dao and applying our knowledge in day-to-day life. The three jewels of Dao are compassion, moderation and humility. The Da Yan or Wild Goose takes us on a journey to find purpose and meaning and to improve our quality of life.

We thank all the previous generations for refining and protecting this ancient healing practice and making it accessible so all can benefit.

# Chapter 2
# Wu Wei
# The Essence of Da Yan Qigong

## Da Yan - Wild Goose Qigong
### The 2nd 64 movements

## Wu Wei – The Essence of Da Yan Qigong

One of the main underlying principles of the Chinese healing arts and the Daoist understanding of life, is the concept of 'Wu Wei'. This translates to 'non-action'; doing things without really doing anything. Unfortunately, in modern society we tend to think too much. This wastes a lot of energy and most of the time is unnecessary. Firstly we need to relax, to calm the mind and just be. Wu Wei is action without desire or motivation. Wu Wei refers to the cultivation of a state of being in which our actions are quite effortless and without even trying, we are able to respond perfectly to whatever situations arise; to simply go with the flow.

The concept of Wu Wei does take time to grasp and integrate into our lives. When we first start our study of Da Yan Wild Goose Qigong there are many movements to learn; it's only through repetitive practice that we are able to remember the sequence. Then we learn the details and integrate them into the practice. The final stage is incorporating the Qi flow once these three levels of training have been achieved, then the understanding of Wu Wei will become more natural. Even in the early stages, students can have small glimpses of the subtleness of Wu Wei as the practice purges the energy system increasing our Qi field. When this happens, the mind and body will find balance and harmony and the concept of Wu Wei will be realised naturally.

**Wu Wei**

*By staying unoccupied and being peaceful*
*You can observe the coming and going of all people and all lives.*

*After reaching prosperity,*
*All lives must know to return to the root.*
*To return to the root is to be still and quiet.*
*This is how the life force is able to return.*

*To return to the root is the function of the subtle path.*
*With clarity*
*You follow the way of the subtle path,*
*and do not wait to become exhausted.*
*Otherwise the life force cannot return.*

*It is dangerous to engage*
*in fanciful and wild behaviour*
*when one does not know the subtle path.*
*By following the normal operation of the subtle path,*
*One becomes receptive.*
*By being receptive,*
*One becomes selfless.*
*By being selfless,*
*One attains spiritual kingship (self mastery).*
*By attaining spiritual kingship,*
*One becomes godly and heavenly*
*(able to connect with god or heaven).*
*By being godly and heavenly,*
*One becomes united with the subtle path.*
*By uniting with the eternity of the subtle path, One's life continues*
*even after the body ceases to exist.*

**Lao Tzu, Dao De Jing, Chapter 16**

Master Chen describes the essence of Da Yan Qigong and how to practise it in order to receive the full benefits of this ancient Chinese healing art: 'The law of nature is used for the exercise of stillness and non-action. The principles of these exercises are genuine, correct, and honest, which means that the heart should be pure without distractions, the movement should be correct without alteration and the bearing should be true without pretence.

'Naturalness, stillness, the harmony between man and nature as well as moral personal character and virtue are at the core of the principles and theory of this Qigong. The basic functional state of nothingness and stillness comes more from the exercise of being empty, rather than being still and relaxed. In this way, its magical effects can be achieved. The exercise of being empty and doing nothing represents the essence of Da Yan Qigong.

'The non-action or Wu Wei in Daoism means that as long as the Dao is not obstructed by any ideas or thoughts, the highest state of nothingness will be attained. Action and non-action are a unity of the opposites, in that something can be created from nothing and nothing comes from something. Therefore, action and non-action are always together. There is non-action in action and action always comes back to non-action, just like the acquired comes back to the innate. It is essential for those who exercise the art to grasp the subtlety in it. The result of action is explicit while the outcome of non-action is implicit. The exercise of non-action is the true meaning.

'When exercising, one should not think anything or use any of his ideas as guidance or to promote his circulation, and this is the exercise of being empty and the exercise of spirit. The spirit includes the primordial spirit, which is the foundation of spirit, and the mental spirit, which is the spirit of thought. Therefore, action originates from the ideas of mental spirit while non-action, from that of the primordial spirit, which is the true idea. The exercise of Qigong is the exercise of mind, or the spirit. As long as one keeps his primordial spirit full and his mental spirit quiet, he is able to promote his energy. If the mental spirit is full but the primordial is short, there will be an opposite effect.

'The Da Yan Qigong features a rigorous system and a scientific structure, with both a harmonious connection to the nature outside and an agreement with the Qi of the human body inside. It means that the key of the Da Yan Qigong is the aura or Qi field as a whole and since the Five Elements and the Eight Diagrams each have their fixed spots within the human body, it is essential that we practise this Qigong exactly according to the requirements for those spots without any change. And if any change should occur, the balance of the Qigong would be destroyed, which would lead to the destruction of its essence. Therefore, the combination of Qi and blood, of muscle and bone, of heart and lung, of internal and external, of Yin and Yang as well as of gesture and ideas, would not be achieved.

'The Da Yan Qigong, created by ancient masters, has been enriched and developed in its more than 1000 years of promotion, thanks to the contribution of the people who inherited and passed on its essence through the ages.'

# Chapter 3
# A Continuing Journey

Da Yan - Wild Goose Qigong
The 2nd 64 movements

☯

# A Continuing Journey

My life changed in 1979 when I had a near-death experience. I have realised for a long time that the tragic accident that I had when was nineteen years of age was a blessing in disguise. I would never have met so many amazing people and had the opportunity to be involved in their healing journeys. I don't like to think about it too much, but it is a major driving motivational force, guiding my life. The realisation of the self or when the 'I' became present is a classical spiritual awakening story. Many before me and many after will have similar experiences. This light within, shining from the realisation of the self, has stayed on as I have found a cultivation path to continue to nurture it.

The Chinese healing arts have helped heal my body, nurture my mind and cultivate my spirit. I have been fortunate in that I have had the opportunity to teach and lead many groups; all of us are on a journey of self-discovery. Through experience we gain wisdom and this acceptance that we all have wisdom can actively aid in the development of ourselves and our community, which helps to keep the spiritual light turned on. According to the Dao, which means the source or the fresh pure energy of the universe and of all life, virtue is the highest reality. Virtue grows and develops from wisdom. Virtue is a way of living in accord with life's rules. Virtue is what maintains us and ensures calmness and peace.

When I started studying the Chinese healing arts I gained a lot of knowledge by learning many different forms or styles. This was very important as it takes time to grasp the basics, develop a strong structure of the physical movements and to open the energy channels. There are many good quality teachers who can guide you to this point, but if you want to go further you need to put the work in and master as much as you can yourself, then seek out specialist teachers or masters in the areas that you are interested in.

I started travelling to China regularly from 1998, attending international Qigong conferences and leading study groups. Here I was exposed to many different traditional and newer styles of Qigong. My main interest was cultivating the Dao. I cut back and stopped teaching and practising the internal martial Qigong styles (Taijiquan) and felt guided to different teachers. My earlier books *Absorbing the Essence* and *Restoring Natural Harmony* document these experiences studying Daoist and medical Qigong. To cultivate the Dao we need to work on and develop ourselves, so we can ultimately achieve true knowledge from our own firsthand experiences.

I started leading study groups to China not only to learn Qigong and to absorb the ancient culture, but mainly to connect with the Qi at the sacred mountains and holy temples. Through history, many pilgrims and spiritual seekers have travelled to these sacred places to increase their knowledge and cultivate wisdom and virtue. I received formal Daoist training from Grand Master Zhong Yunlong at Wudang Mountain in 1999 and 2000, but being non-Chinese, it can be difficult to be taken seriously and treated as any more than a general tourist when visiting these sacred places.

I'm fortunate that my good friend and study tour partner Zhang Jing helped me enormously in making it possible to get to these out-of-the-way places and translating to the main people my purpose for being there. On the 2005 study tour we were visiting Qufu in Shandong province, the hometown of Confucius. Earlier in the day I had seen a Daoist priest also visiting one of the temples. Jing and I were walking through the Confucius Forest which is a beautiful garden that has a special energy and where Confucius's burial mound or tomb is kept. As we were walking we bumped into the Daoist priest. I acknowledged him with a special greeting that Grand Master Zhong had showed me. It's a way of holding the hands together to form a Yin/Yang shape making an energy connection with another Daoist. Master Xiang Li was impressed with my greeting and enquired from Jing who I was. We struck up an instant friendship; Master Xiang Li was from a neighbouring province and buying new tiles for the monastery he was reconstructing. He invited me to bring a group and visit him at his monastery. The next year, on the 2006 study tour, we went to the Immortal Platform and stayed at the White Cloud Temple as guests of Master Xiang Li.

The Immortal Platform is the site of an ancient Daoist monastery in Hubei province in central China. We had planned on a two night stay to visit Master Xiang Li. It was a long journey into the countryside and it took four hours to find our way there by bus and another hour to walk up the mountain, as the road was too steep for the bus to drive. When we finally arrived, Master Xiang Li welcomed us as the first foreign group to visit this remote temple nestled up high in the mountains. He told us a German man once visited in the1930s. Master Xiang Li spent quality time with our group discussing Daoist ideas and sharing healing techniques. We had to leave the next day as it took us longer than expected to get there and we had to go back to Wuhan the capital of Hubei province to get a train connection to continue our journey.

**Immortal Platform**

**Grand Master Cheng Zhen, Changchun - Eternal Spring Monastery, Wuhan**

Master Xiang Li rang his Daoist brother at the Eternal Spring Monastery in Wuhan to introduce us and welcome us for a visit when we were in Wuhan. I had heard of the Changchung or Eternal Spring Monastery; it's a large monastery with a history of over 2000 years and I was pleased that we were going to visit. We were welcomed by the assistant abbott and personally shown around. Jing translated and we learned about the history of the monastery and Dragon Gate Daoism and taken to different shrine rooms, learning about the importance of each one. Finally we were led to a tea room where we sat and were served delicious green tea. A Daoist nun joined us and she sat in a lotus position (cross-legged) staring at us with a big beautiful smile. I asked Jing who she was and he replied that she was the abbott and that she liked our energy. We spent an hour with Grand Master Cheng Zhen. She wanted to know all about us so Jing told her about the different members of our group and the type of work that I do and the purpose of our travel to China. When we left she said that we were welcome to come back to Wuhan and study Daoism with her.

The following year in 2007 I organised a group studying Guigen Qigong to practise with Dr Xu Hongtao in Beijing. We arranged a side trip to Wuhan for one week to study with Grand Master Cheng Zhen. We went to the monastery each morning. Grand Master Cheng Zhen would discuss the Daoist understanding of life and ways of incorporating the Dao into our lives; we spent a lot of the time in meditation 'returning to nothingness'. Many of her other students came to meet us and after four days she asked me if we would like to become her students and be initiated at the monastery. A few days later, a large ceremony was arranged and all of our group became a 25th Generation of Dragon Gate Daoism including my new Daoist brother Jing. We all received Daoist names; my initiated name is 'Xin Si' which means 'Genuine Wisdom'. It was a special time for all of us and it was during this time of high energy connection that I met Grand Master Chen, the 28th generation lineage holder of the Da Yan Wild Goose Qigong.

I have been back up the mountain a few times to visit Master Xiang Li at the Immortal Platform and I also visit Wuhan at least once or twice a year. Each time I visit the Eternal Spring Monastery to see Grand Master Cheng Zhen or my other Daoist brothers. We have even had a few meetings with both Grand Masters of the Dao and Da Yan Wild Goose Qigong together.

**Initiation**

When we study Qigong we first learn the form or shape of the movements. Then we study the details and then the Qi or energy flow from the external to the internal. There are many different styles and some of the basic principles apply to most styles. However, some styles have their own special training methods and it's important not to overlap one Qigong training method with another; not to mix styles and create hybrid forms as this can cause problems. There are many good teachers who can instruct the movements, share the details and give you an understanding of the Qi flow. But, for the serious student who wants to learn more of the details and fully understand and cultivate their Qi, it's advisable to become initiated into a lineage. This traditional process can take time as the student needs to show that they are of good moral character and possesses an open and caring heart. Once the student has shown all these qualities, then generally a special ceremony is performed where the student will recite special values and sometimes the Master will touch or even hit (slap) the new student to transmit the energy of the lineage.

There are many newer styles of Chinese exercises being developed and promoted in recent times and while there are many benefits, some have lost their true meaning and energy connection by simply becoming another 'mindful' gentle exercise. The first style of the Chinese healing arts that I learned was a modified Yang Style Taijiquan (Tai Chi Chuan). I became an instructor with this organisation and began to teach, but over time I became disillusioned and then sought out more traditional styles (this story is told in my first book *The Art of Life*). I eventually became an initiated student of Tai Chi Master William Ho in Sydney. Master Ho is very proud of his family's lineage both his parents were martial artists and his grandfather was a disciple of Yang Cheng Pu, one of the Yang family's Taijiquan Grand Masters. I have always had great respect for my teachers and have tried to pass on their cultural and healing legacies. I only teach Qigong styles that have been directly transmitted and taught to me and that I have been given authority to teach. I have my own style of teaching, but I have never invented my own style of Qigong.

During the Chinese summer of 2010, when I received my first private training of the Da Yan Wild Goose Qigong with Grand Master Chen in Wuhan, the Master and Madam mentioned the possibility of becoming an initiated student. I told them I was interested and from then on I met many of their other family members and senior students who wanted to know all about my family history and my plans for the future.

In the following year, the training was held at a smaller town called Luyi in Henan province. Luyi is a very sacred place as it's the birthplace and hometown of Lao Tzu, one of the Great Masters of the Dao. I took three of my senior students, all qualified Qigong teachers, and we were joined by Master and Madam Chen and a few of their senior students from nearby provinces. The Master and Madam have visited Luyi many times and there is a large group of Da Yan Wild Goose Qigong students there. It was also a favourite training spot for Grand Master Yang Mei Jung, Master Chen's mother.

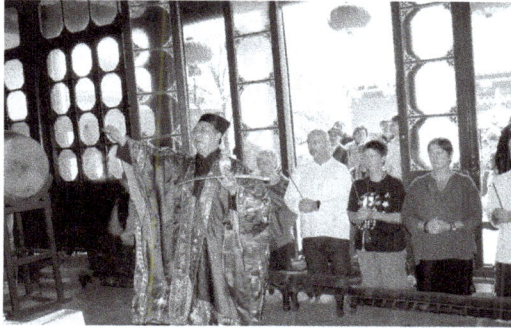

**Initiation Ceremony Dragon Gate Daoism
Eternal Spring Monastery, Wuhan**

**Initiation Ceremony Dragon Gate Daoism
Eternal Spring Monastery, Wuhan**

**Initiation Ceremony, Da Yan Wild Goose Qigong, Wuhan**

**Initiation Ceremony, Da Yan Wild Goose Qigong, Wuhan**

There are many sacred temples and historical places there, all with a special energy. We would practise every day with the local group and absorb this precious energy. We had many discussions with Daoist masters which helped us gain a deeper understanding of the principles of the Dao; it was a special time of growth for all of us. We filmed a DVD with Grand Master Chen leading our group in both the 1st and 2nd 64 movement sets in the grounds of the Ming Dao Temple. The following year in 2012, I was accepted as an initiated student and a large ceremony was held in Wuhan and I became a 29th generation of the Da Yan Wild Goose Qigong.

When travelling to China with study groups we visit many sacred Daoist areas. I like to go to the mountains which have a special Qi field that we can connect with to help improve our own Qi field. I have been fortunate that I have visited these places many times, receiving special blessings from the masters at monasteries and temples. One such place is called 'Qing Cheng Shan' translating to 'Green City Mountain' in Sichuan Province in south west China. We have visited here many times, staying at the guest house at the Heavenly Masters Cave. Grand Master Tang Cheng Qing is the abbott; his cultivation practice is mainly through meditation and Chinese painting. Master Tang specialises in four traditional paintings of the four seasons and on each trip he has painted one for me transmitting his Qi into each one. These four paintings of Bamboo, Orchids, Chrysanthemums and Plum Blossoms are known as 'The Four Noble Ones' and are said to show virtues of an honourable man (based on the teaching of Confucius). I have presented them with his permission in the four books that I have written about my training experiences in China.

**Bamboo** refers to the season of summer. The tall, straight stems symbolise honour and nobility, while the hollow stalks represent humility, tranquillity and inner peace. Also the flexibility and strength of the bamboo stalk symbolises the values of cultivation and integrity in which one yields but does not break. The Bamboo is featured in the book *Absorbing the Essence*, presenting the Daoist cultivation practices taught to me at Wudang Mountain.

**Orchid** refers to the season of spring. The beauty and grace of the orchid represents integrity, nobility and friendship. Great scholars aspired to these qualities of the orchid to form a good educational background, to be humble yet elegant, be natural yet refined and independent yet friendly. Orchids are featured in the book *Restoring Natural Harmony* which presents Chinese medical Qigong and Guigen Qigong taught to me at the Xiyuan Hospital in Beijing.

**Chrysanthemum** refers to the season of autumn. The blazing colour of flowering chrysanthemums as the weather turns cooler symbolises the virtue to withstand all adversities; to challenge all difficulties and to maintain nobility and elegance while striving to create a better life. Chrysanthemums are featured in the book *Da Yan Wild Goose Qigong- the 1st 64 movements*.

**Plum Blossom** refers to the season of winter. The full flowering blossoms in winter resemble a fierce dragon and represents endurance and perseverance as well as symbolising inner beauty and humility under adverse conditions. They represent new ideas and creativity and striving to create new inventions to improve the human race. Plum Blossoms are featured in the book *Da Yan Wild Goose Qigong- The 2nd 64 movements.*

As a teacher all I can do is give the facts. It's up to the individual to process this information and make it their own. It's important to take time out for ourselves each day, to practise both movement and meditation in order to balance the internal Qi with the external Qi to make it whole. This allows our body's functions to run smoothly, our mind to find peace and our spirit to rise. As we grow older our Qi diminishes, but Qi can be developed and transformed into a higher, more subtle kind of energy called Shen which is the spiritual level of energy and is immortal.

Heavenly Masters Cave, Qing Cheng Shan Green City Mountain

**Grand Master, Tang Cheng Qing, Orchid 2004**

**Grand Master, Tang Cheng Qing, Bamboo 2007**

**Grand Master, Tang Cheng Qing
Chrysanthemums and Plum Blossoms 2013**

# Chapter 4
## The Art of Practice

Da Yan - Wild Goose Qigong
The 2nd 64 movements

☯

# The Art of Practice *(this section is repeated from the 1st 64 movement Da Yan Wild Goose book)*

To get the most out of your practice there are a few basic principles and guidelines as well as precautions that you should be aware of. These principles are important for gaining a deeper understanding and realising the full benefits of this ancient healing art. Proper practice ensures positive results and eliminates potential negative effects.

Relaxation and tranquillity are the fundamental requirements and methods for Qigong practice. From the external to the internal, we first start by relaxing the physical body as this helps relieve respiratory and mental tension. Tranquillity means allowing the mind to be calm and find inner peace; the practice of tranquillity in Qigong requires quiet external surroundings and a peaceful internal world. Internal tranquillity, with your mind relaxed and focused, is more important than external silence. Relaxing can induce tranquillity while tranquillity helps relaxing. Complete relaxation is possible only when complete tranquillity is present.

Correct practice helps induce the effect of relaxation and tranquillity, whereas incorrect postures may inhibit one's ability to realise this state of relaxation and tranquillity. Correct postures and movements take time to master and are dependent on the individual's specific physiological and psychological characteristics at their stage of practice. The difficulty and intensity of practice should be adjusted according to the person, the time, the place and their attained state, in order to produce the desired mental and physical relaxation. Otherwise, improper practice may produce only stress and fatigue.

Making it a pleasurable experience as you progress from beginner to advanced level, is a fundamental principle in learning Qigong. We should practice persistently over a long period of time; Qigong practice is a process of constant accumulation. As long as one perseveres with the practice, the effects will be obtained gradually and naturally. Some students show significant improvements within a short period of time, whereas some practitioners do not display any distinctive changes for a long time, and some may start with positive effects which soon diminish. Whatever the effects, it is important to have a correct and positive attitude. Being confident about oneself and persistent in practice are important. Qigong is a practical method, and long-term practice is the only way to get real effects. It's common to experience different sensations when practising Qigong. Feeling warmth and a tingling sensation in different parts of the body is common, as well as the rising of emotions and some people even report seeing different colours and visions. Try not to have too much attention on sensations as it can deplete your Qi experience. It's better to go to the level of no sensation to return to nothingness.

**The Philosophy of the Wild Goose**
The wild goose is a high energy bird which flies thousands of kilometres from one side of the world to the other and over 10 000 meters high up over the mountains. It is very graceful, as well as being proud and honourable. It's also very protective of its flock. When we practise we try to adopt some of these characteristics, as this will increase our Qi field and make practice more enjoyable.

In ancient Chinese and Egyptian cultures the wild goose was considered a messenger between heaven and earth. In India the wild goose is known as the 'vahana' or the vehicle for which Brahma the Hindu God of creation travels on. It's also associated with the sun, prana (Qi), knowledge, atman, spirit and the creation of life itself. In China, geese are still a symbol of marriage and long life; in rural communities a newly married couple would be given a pair of geese as a wedding present to signify their bond of marriage. In the Roman Empire, the wild goose was the sacred animal of Juno, the protector of women and the goddess of light, marriage and childbirth.

The Ganalbingu or the Magpie Goose people, the ancient indigenous inhabitants of central Arnhem Land Australia, have lived in harmony with their land and environment for thousands of years. The goose, their eggs and their nests are sacred to the Ganalbingu people. Special ceremonies depicting the goose are held for aiding the health of newborn babies and their mothers.

The goose, with its powerful flight and migratory habits, can be associated with travelling. The journey may be difficult, but the goose can help people find perseverance. In earlier times, shamans were aided by spirit geese on their journeys to other worlds. In modern psychotherapy geese are associated with communication or the ability to express oneself. In ancient mythology as in modern psychotherapy, geese are still regarded as symbols of marriage and the importance of a solid, happy home and family life.

During the 1st 64 movement set the goose is resting in between journeys; its feeding and gathering energy preparing for its next flight. In the opening movements we have an image of these birds being happy and having fun. The purpose of these movements is to gather good Qi from all directions and to disperse bad Qi. To become one with the universe. The goose is flying over water (lakes and rivers) and it is feeling happy. It looks for good Qi from the distance, for pure Qi; grasping it for increased energy and preparing for its next journey. Playing with the Qi ball brings good Qi into the body. Then the goose descends as it looks for water and food. It continues to process and refine Qi after its all-day activity, then it finds its way back to the nest before dark and goes to sleep. During the 2nd 64 movement set the goose awakens in the morning and calls on the rest of the flock to embark on a great flying journey. It still exercises during the flight to regain energy; it gathers good Qi through its eyes from looking at the sun, moon and Milky Way.

**The Five Aspects of Naturalness**
When practising, Grand Master Chen advises that we follow the five requirements of naturalness:

1. **The naturalness of mind.** 'Exercise with no guidance from the mind. Have a free and empty mind without deliberately clearing it, because it can always be clear as long as no attention is paid to it.'
2. **The naturalness of breath.** 'There is no need to regulate the breath. Just follow its natural flow. The breath will be regulated after the aura or Qi field is open and clear.'
3. **The naturalness of body.** 'Keep the knees straight in a natural and relaxed way. Relax the face and let down the shoulders and elbows. Relax the waist and hip and keep the chest slightly open without folding it or humping the back. Clear the Ren channel and lift the back to let the Du channel run smoothly.'
4. **The naturalness of metabolism.** 'With the mechanism of exercises, the stale Qi inside can be exhaled from the body and the primordial Qi, or Yuan Qi can be inhaled so that the acupoints and the channels can be cleared and the aura or Qi field can also be motivated. As a result, the internal organs can be nourished, which will speed up the process of the merging of the natural Qi and the primordial Qi in the body.'
5. **The naturalness of exercise.** 'Keep a relaxed and quiet state of mind. There is no need to pretend, as the right state of mind will come during the exercise. Place the tip of the tongue on the roof of the mouth to link the Ren and the Du channel and let the body fluid flow back down to the diaphragm. Keep the eyes steady with the light outside and the spirit inside. As a result, there will come the state of emptiness and the Qi outside will naturally be inhaled. And at this moment the mind will follow the movement, which is the so-called unity of movement and mind. All the movements from the start to the end of the exercise make up the cycle of motivation, circulation, enhancing and gathering of the vital Qi inside the body, which will bring a great balance and an overall effect to the function of the body. The naturalness of exercise also means that the Da Yan Qigong is suitable for people of all ages.'

## The health and healing benefits

There are many health and healing benefits associated with regular practice of the Da Yan Wild Goose Qigong. Within the instruction sections of the 1st and 2nd 64 movement books, both the anatomical and energetic benefits for each movement are listed. Theoretically each individual movement will benefit a specific area or condition, but it is the accumulation of practising the complete set of exercises from the beginning to the end many times, when the real benefits will be realised. From my own experience and the feedback that I have received from my students, the many bending, twisting and stretching movements aid in blood circulation, flexibility and balance as well as overall strengthening of the whole body. Please read the inspiring stories sections in both books, telling of individual's own experiences of practising these Chinese healing arts for many years.

## Meditation, processing the Qi

Our thinking mind uses the most energy of our body; when the mind is calm and relaxed it can increase our energy, whereas when the mind is very active it can deplete our energy. After practising the dynamic moving sections of the Da Yan Wild Goose Qigong, we practise the static or stillness section. This part of our practice is very important; when the body comes to a complete stop, the Qi keeps moving and through the tranquillity of the mind, the Qi will come into order. It's what we call the 'processing' stage; it's important to keep your thinking mind out of the way and to allow the Qi to do its work. The movements clear the meridian system, dispelling stale Qi and absorbing good Qi, helping foster Yang with tranquillity breeding Yin. To balance Yin and Yang we need a good balance between dynamic and static; too much movement or stillness by itself can unbalance Yin and Yang.

## Where and when to practise

The wild goose always flies the same route so it can find its way home again. So try to do your practice at the same time and at the same place. The goose is fussy and choosey when coming back to the nest. It likes to make it cosy for a good night's sleep, ready for the next day's journey. Practising in one regular location will create and form a Qi field and this will improve your Qi development. I remember one time we were practising with Grand Master Chen before breakfast and it was raining and we couldn't go outside to our regular spot. We found a spot under cover near the hotel and Master Chen led us in Goose Walking; we walked around in a circle with our arms away from our body similar to the commencing movement for a few minutes. This created a Qi field on our new practice area; once we had cleansed the space we began to practise.

It's important when we start our practice to face towards the western direction if this is possible; this is because the structure of the movements are based on the Five Elements. The different directions relate to the elements and their corresponding meridians and organ groups of the body. The Da Yan Wild Goose set moves in all directions while absorbing the Qi from the Five Elements and the universe. This accumulative effect builds the Qi in the body. There are many stepping and walking types of movements used for balancing Yin and Yang; each time the foot presses the earth it is Yin and each time it releases it is Yang.

When we start as new students, it's important to practise with a group, as the flock works together to help each other. This group energy also creates a strong Qi field that everyone benefits from. Another way is to attend regular retreats and intensive training sessions, which also increases your Qi field. In time we can practise on our own to master the movements and make them our own.

Exercising in the early morning and late afternoon when the sun rises and sets is a very powerful time, as there is a natural transition between the dark coolness of night (Yin) and the bright warmth of day (Yang). The setting of the sun and transition between Yang and Yin is also a time when nature has a great influence on your body. You might notice that birds are very active at this time of day, as they are in the morning. It's important not to look directly into the sun in the early morning or late afternoon, as this can cause damage to your eyes.

Qigong can be practised anywhere, but some places are better than others. You should be undisturbed during Qigong practice to help maintain concentration in the mind. The best places are in nature in the open air where the heaven (Yang) and earth (Yin) Qi are most abundant. Practise in the mountains or beside a waterfall or the ocean; near water is excellent because moving water generates a lot of Qi.

If you are practising indoors, try to find a quiet and peaceful space away from draughts with natural light and fresh air. Avoid excessive noise, TV sets and computers and turn off your mobile phone or set it to silent.

The proximity of some plants should also be avoided. The Oleander plant for example, is known to be poisonous and has a very tense Qi. As you practice you will learn which plants feel relaxing and harmonious. Lovely flowers and large old trees are ideal.

As a rule, you should not exercise on a full or empty stomach. Instead of eating breakfast, consume liquids as they stimulate stomach-intestine movement which acts as an internal massage. Warm or room temperature water is the best with a slice of lemon, but not cold water from the fridge, as this interferes with Qi circulation.

Qigong exercise in the evenings is a way of freeing your mind and body from the burdens of a busy day; a way of processing the events of the day and letting things go, physically and emotionally. Students often comment on how they get their best night's sleep after attending class. You are able to sleep more quietly and recover more fully because the body begins its recovery during Qigong and this continues during sleep.

We are all a bit different, so I wouldn't advise anyone practising just before going to sleep as it stimulates your energy and may disrupt your sleep. But a few students have told me that when they haven't been able to sleep, they would get up and practise Qigong to calm their mind and body, then have a restful sleep afterwards.

## Eating and drinking

For Qigong exercise you need a clear head. Beverages such as alcohol, tea and coffee affect concentration and your body's functions. If you are not calm and relaxed you will not feel the full benefits from Qigong exercise. It's best to avoid drinking cold fluids during or immediately after practice as this interferes with Qi circulation.

You should not exercise on either an empty stomach or after a full meal. Being distracted by hunger will not help your mental focus, so if you are hungry have something light to eat or something to drink. A full stomach interferes with Qi circulation. The Qi is diverted into the digestive system as stomach juices increase and stomach-intestinal movements occur, leaving very little Qi to circulate elsewhere.

## When not to exercise

When we exercise we absorb the good influences from nature and the macrocosm. Similarly, we assimilate the influences from turbulent weather conditions. Therefore, it is not good to practise Qigong during bad weather, heavy fog, extreme heat, before or during a thunderstorm, on excessively windy days, or during lunar or solar eclipses. Exercise can begin again when nature is balanced.

## Menstruation and pregnancy

Qigong is good to practice during menstruation and pregnancy as it will improve the circulation of Qi, blood and other bodily fluids.

Women who are menstruating should pay attention to the effects of Qigong exercise. If the exercise produces a negative effect, stop immediately and continue at a later time.

Special care is also required during pregnancy. Each woman's pregnancy is different and it is recommended that the expectant mother consult her primary care provider as well as a qualified and experienced Qigong teacher.

## What to wear

There are no rules regarding clothing but since relaxation is important in Qigong, try to wear loose comfortable clothing, ideally made of natural fibres such as cotton or silk.

If you are limited in what you can wear, for example if you are at work, loosen your collar and tie, your belt or waistband and remove uncomfortable or high heeled shoes. It's important that you wear flat soled shoes or even bare feet are OK. I always wear soft sports shoes as I damaged my feet and ankles a long time ago and I find wearing shoes gives me a bit more support. It's a personal preference and there are many light soft shoes available that are suitable.

Whatever clothing you choose to wear, it should not be tight around the waist because the Qi needs to flow easily. Preferably, remove watches and bracelets as they restrict the flow of Qi through the wrist.

If it is chilly, dress appropriately. Feeling cold during a Qigong session can decrease the effectiveness of the exercises, particularly if your hands, stomach or back are cold; chilling your kidneys severely restricts your Qi circulation. I often start my practice on colder mornings with gloves, hat and a warm jacket; you can always take them off when you heat up.

## How long to practise

The benefits that are gained from Qigong are proportional to the amount of practice undertaken. The Da Yan Wild Goose Qigong 1st 64 movement set takes approximately ten minutes to complete. It is recommended practising three times through, for a total of thirty minutes at least once a day. It is only when the body's carriage is regulated according to Qigong principles that the Qi will flow easily and the benefits of Qigong realised. If you can achieve thirty minutes twice a day, you will notice a marked increase in vitality and peace within a few weeks. If you have major health issues and can manage a couple of hours per day, you will soon see a radical improvement in your health and wellbeing. Regardless of your state of health when you begin, any amount of regular practice will improve how you feel.

The 2nd 64 movement set of Da Yan Wild Goose Qigong also takes approximately ten minutes to complete. When you are comfortable and have mastered both the 1st and 2nd 64 movement sets, Grand Master Chen advises that we practise the 1st 64 movement set twice, followed by the 2nd 64 movement set once, for a total of thirty minutes twice a day.

**How long does the effect of Qigong exercise last?**

Qigong works because the Qi is brought into order and the mind, body and spirit are in harmony. This harmony can be disturbed by arguing, getting excited or annoyed, engaging in strenuous physical activity, eating excessively and even going to the toilet. If possible, use the toilet beforehand rather than after Qigong exercise because urination and defecation bring the Qi into definite motion.

I often tell my students after a Qigong class that if they have driven a car there not to play the radio when they leave, as all your senses have been enhanced and the body functions are in harmony. You may get good ideas, solve some problems or if you are with friends you may have amazing conversations. Look at the beauty of the sky, trees and the divine in all living things; I love to look at clouds. It's a creative time, so use it and the Qi will be with you longer. The more you cultivate your Qi the more in harmony with the universe you will be, improving all aspects of your life.

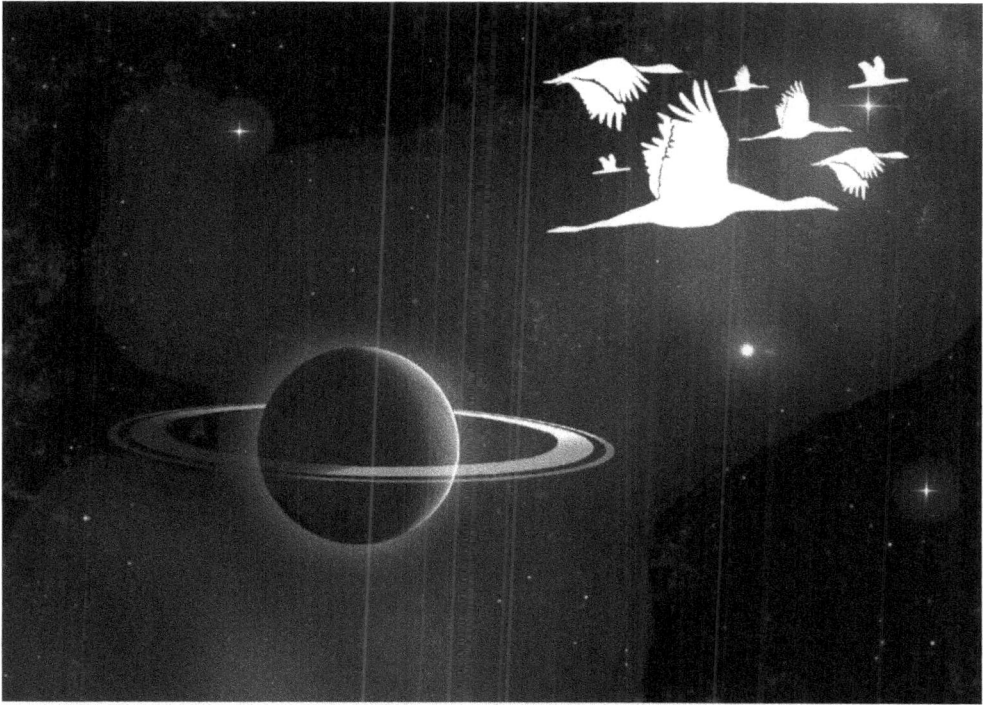

# Chapter 5
# Qigong Preparation

Da Yan - Wild Goose Qigong

The 2nd 64 movements

# Qigong Preparation

Qigong is a cultivation exercise which benefits the physical body, the energetic or Qi body as well as the mind. It allows us to rebalance our mind, body and breath and with regular practice it enables us to create a healthy lifestyle and to identify our true spiritual nature.

It is important to create the right conditions before, during and after practice to get the best results. According to the ancient Daoist way of understanding our relationship and connection with the universe, we allow our internal landscape to harmonise with the external landscape.

Da Yan Wild Goose Qigong is a very dynamic set of movements with a lot of bending and stretching. It is important to prepare the mind, body and breath before we start to practise. Qigong practices abide by the basic principles of the three adjustments or three tunings. It is a way of calming the mental activity of the brain and turning on and tuning the mind to tune into the breath and the body.

- **Tuning the Mind**
- **Tuning the Breath**
- **Tuning the Body**

Qigong should never be practised when you are feeling physically cold, energetically cold or emotionally cold. The Qi will not flow very well and can even have an adverse or harmful effect. Good preparation is equally as important as good practice and a good close.

The warm-up is not only a way of preparing the mind and body for the Qigong movements that follow, it is also very good exercise. Physically, when we loosen and rotate the joints, we exercise the ligaments and tendons as well as the membranes which secrete synovial fluid to lubricate the joints. This can improve many arthritic conditions. Energetically, we clear stagnant energy (Qi) that can accumulate around the joints. The stretching movements also help stimulate the meridian system as well as strengthen the muscular system. According to Traditional Chinese Medicine (TCM), the Qi draws the blood through the body. So when we stimulate the Qi circulation we also stimulate blood circulation.

Generally, when we have finished the warm-up, we feel warm, tingling and have turned on and tuned into the body, breath and mind.

# Preparing the mind

During the preparation and warm-up we first concentrate on the mind and allow the excess Yang energy or activity of the brain to descend down. When we have too much activity in this area it can be very hard to concentrate. We keep our mind in the present moment by initially concentrating on the flow of the breath. In time the breath will become smooth and even and this will allow your mind to rest.

When we are in this relaxed state we can use our intention and direct our awareness, like the light of a torch, on each part of the body as we are exercising it, from head to toe. Through this active meditation we consciously awaken the body by feeling and seeing what we are doing.

# Preparing the posture and breath

Keep the body upright with the head and spine naturally in alignment; allow the muscles and flesh to relax around the skeleton. The movements of Qigong help clear the energy blockages in our body. With time and practice the movements will become natural and effortless.

There are a number of different breathing patterns for different styles of Qigong. For the styles presented here, we will breathe in and out through the nose to the abdominal area, slowly, deeply and naturally. When we breathe in, the abdomen gently expands and when breathing out, it gently contracts. This is known as natural breathing. In time, the breath will naturally coordinate with the movements, helping the mind to focus and allowing a fusion between mind, body and breath.

# Basic stance

Stand with feet parallel, shoulder-width apart, as if standing on train tracks, with the knees slightly off lock. Let your weight sink into your legs, feet and into the ground. Keep the coccyx or tail bone slightly tucked in, chest relaxed, and the back straight. Hold your arms away from the body. Fingers are open and relaxed and pointing to the earth; palms are facing the body.

With the chin slightly tucked in and the top of the head (Bai Hui point) reaching to the sky as if a silken cord attached to it is lifting the whole body, lift the Hui Yin, gently squeezing the pelvic floor. Relax your eyes and face and look out into the distance. Keeping your jaw relaxed, place the tip of your tongue on the top palate of your mouth, just behind the front teeth. Breathe in and out through the nose. When breathing in, let the abdomen push out slightly and as the breath goes out, let the abdomen come in. Just relax, letting the whole body breathe.

With the eyes closed, allow the breath to become smooth and even, and let your mind rest. After a few breaths, concentrate on the out-breath, relaxing from the top of the head to the soles of the feet. Just relax down through the body on the out-breath. After a few more breaths, let the knees and hips sink a bit closer to the ground, feel the pressure go into the feet. Like a tree, follow the roots from the soles of your feet deeply into the ground. As you let the breath out, relax down through the body into the ground, letting the stress and tension of the body dissolve into the earth.

After another few breaths, with your awareness, push up the spine one vertebra at a time, checking that the chin tucks in a bit and letting the head pull away from the body. We seem to stand taller as the top of the head reaches up and touches the sky. Stay in this posture for a few breaths, feeling the peace. With your eyes gradually opening, look out into the distance, but not looking.

# The Warm-Up Movements

## Arm and chest stretch

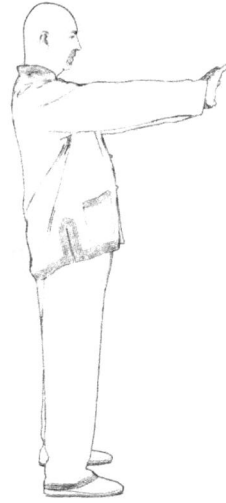

**1a**

**1a (side view)**

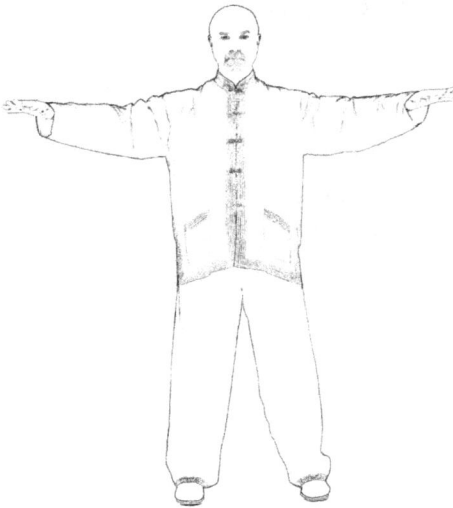

**1b**

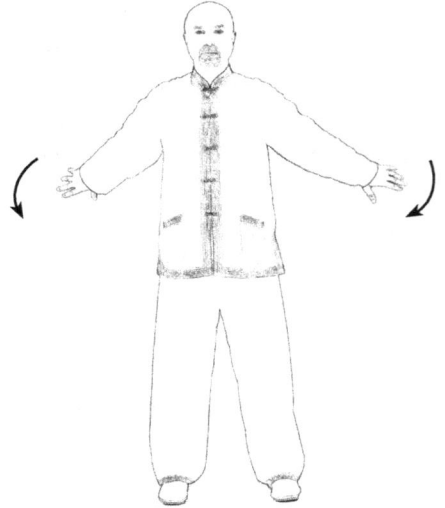

**1c**

**1a-c**  Raise both arms up in front of the body to about shoulder height. Turn your palms out and push to the sides, feeling your chest and rib cage open. Push back and stretch back as far as comfortable.

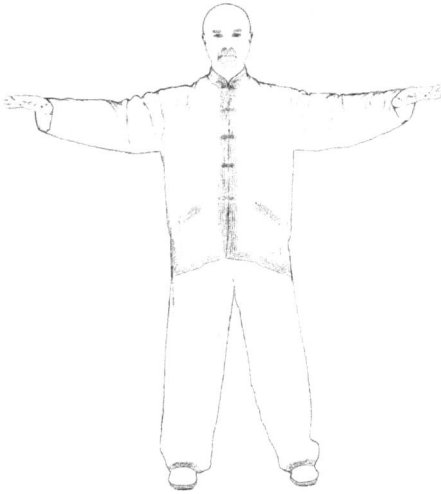

**1d (side view)**                    **1e**                    **1f**

**1d-f**   Turn your palms up, bend the elbows and bring hands to the front of body brushing by the waist. Repeat 4 times, similar to swimming breaststroke.

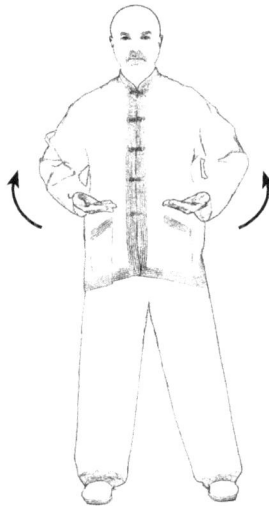
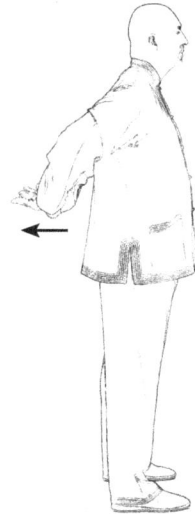

**1g**                    **1h**                    **1i (side view)**

**1g-i**   Then repeat four times in the opposite direction: with palms up, hands brush by your waist and stretch behind; slowly rotate palms and bring arms in front of the body.

This movement exercises the chest, shoulders, elbows and wrists.

# Body roll

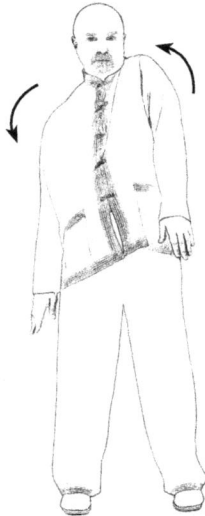

**2a**          **2b**

**2a-b**    Let your arms slowly descend to your sides. Slowly roll one shoulder and then the other, like swimming backstroke. With your awareness, feel the motion massage your shoulders, chest, your abdomen, and your back over the kidney area.

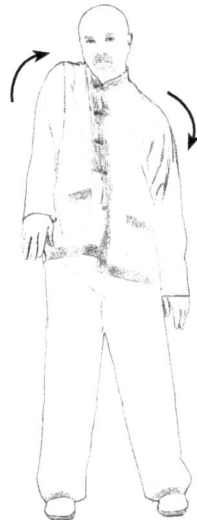

**2c**          **2d**

**2c-d**    After about 8 rotations, stop and come back the other way, rotating forward, and feel the internal massage.

# Hip rotations

**3a**                    **3b**                    **3c**

**3a-c**    Place your hands on your waist and start to move your hips from side-to-side. Relax and feel the movement of the hips.

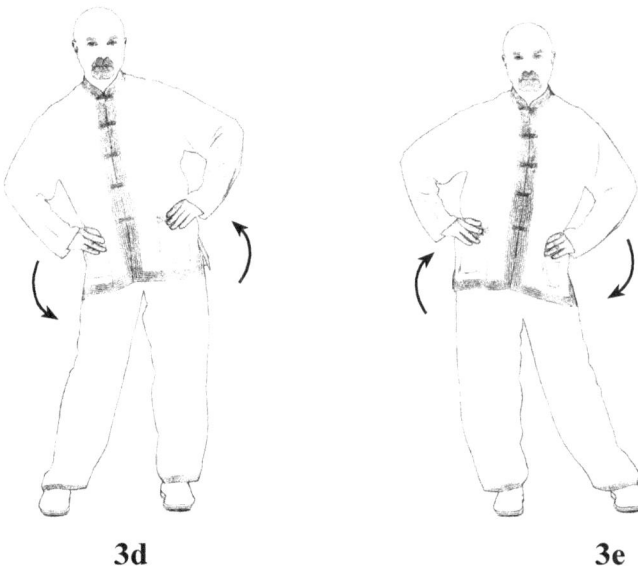

**3d**                              **3e**

**3d-e**    After about three movements to each side, start to move the hips in a circle, gradually increasing your range of movement. Follow the spiralling movement up the spine to the top of your head. Feel and see the movement of the hips. After about 6 rotations, stop and come back the other way.

# Walking and massaging the feet

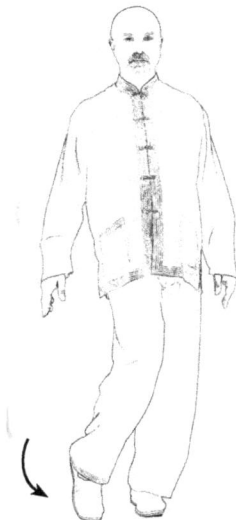

**4a (side view)**          **4b**

**4a-b**   Stand with your feet closer together, walking on the spot. Push firmly from the toe to the heel six times to each side, letting the weight of the body massage the feet. Feel and see the tendons, muscles and joints of the feet.

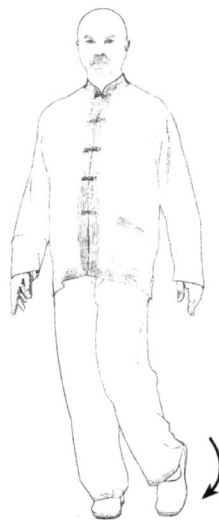

**4c**                    **4d**

**4c-d**    Turn and twist while moving your knee across the body, massaging the inside of the foot on the floor towards the big toe. Repeat about six times to each side.

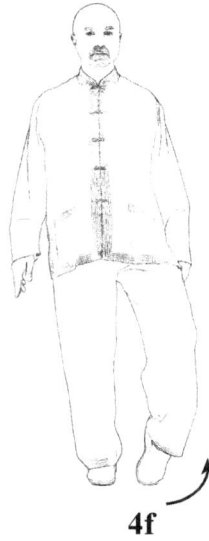

**4e**      **4f**

**4e-f**   Stop and push to the outside of the foot, massaging towards the small toe, 6 to each side. Relax, feel and see the movement of the foot.

## Shaking the legs

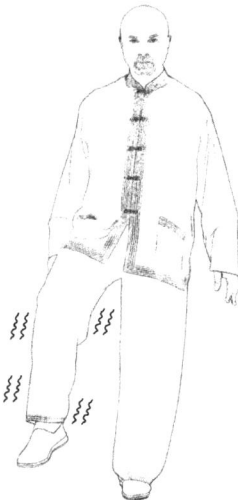
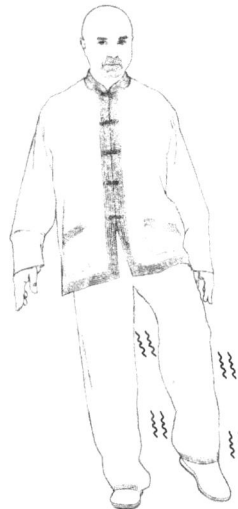

**5a**      **5b**

**5a-b**   Shake your legs three times to each side, allowing the Qi and blood to flow.

# Hand and wrist shaking

**6a-c**     Shake your hands, up and down about 6 times, loosening the hands.

# Back and front stretch

With any type of stretching movement always start gently and then gradually increase your range of movement. With time and practise you will be amazed at how your flexibility will increase.

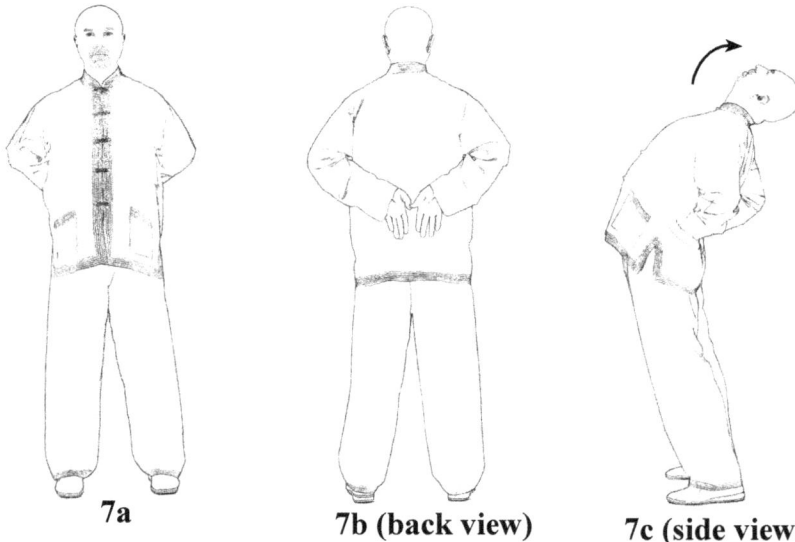

**7a-c**     With your feet parallel, and about shoulder-width apart, place the back of both palms onto your lower back. With your legs straight, gently lean back; only go as far as feels comfortable. With your palms supporting your back, pull your elbows back and gently stretch across your chest and shoulders. Your eyes are looking up towards the sky. With each out-breathe stretch a little more. Continue for a total of four breaths.

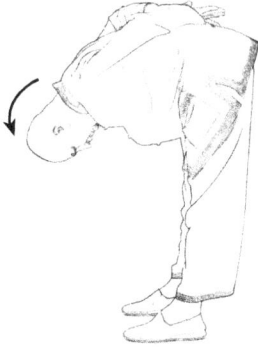 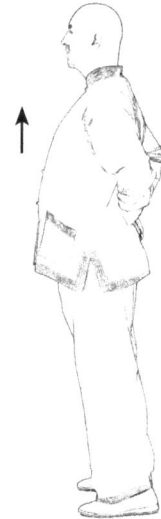

| **7d (side view)** | **7e (side view)** | **7f (side view)** |

**7d-f**  Push your hips back and swing your body forward. Keeping your legs straight and bending from the waist, lean forward and gently fold the body in half. Only go as far as feels comfortable. The eyes are looking between the legs. Gently bend your knees and slowly straighten your back lifting your upper body from the waist. Keeping your shoulders and neck relaxed, with your chin on your chest and eyes looking at the ground. It is important to raise the neck and head last, after the body is upright.

Repeat back and front stretch a total of four times.

# Side stretch

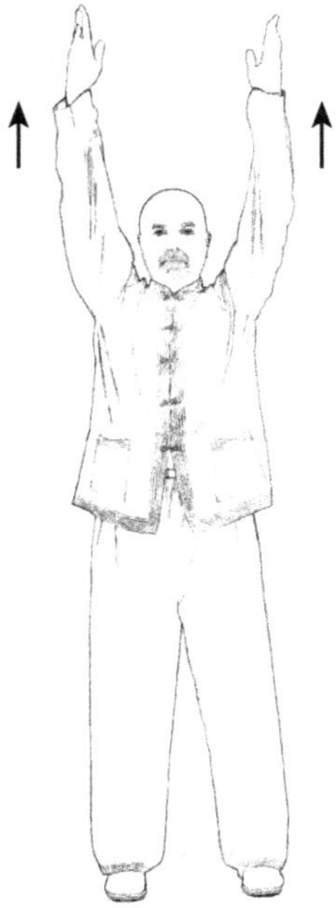

**8a**

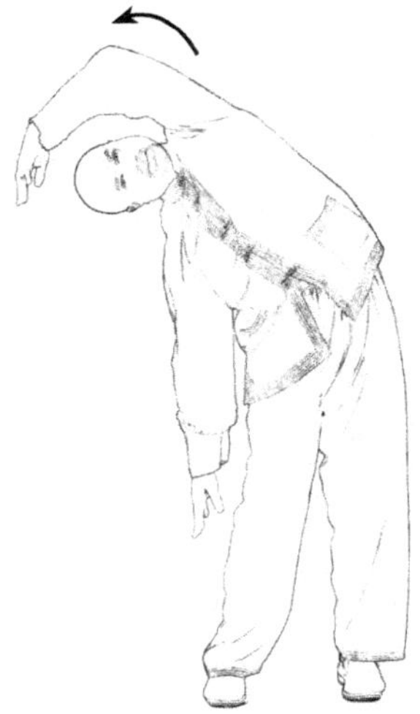

**8b**

**8a**    With feet parallel and about shoulder-width apart, raise both arms up above your head. The palms are facing each other and the fingers are pointing to the sky. Stretch up, lifting your spine.

**8b**    Lower your left arm to the side of your body and lean to your left with your right arm circling over your head; fingers are pointing towards the ground and your eyes are looking towards the sky. With each out breath stretch a little bit more. Continue for a total of four breaths.

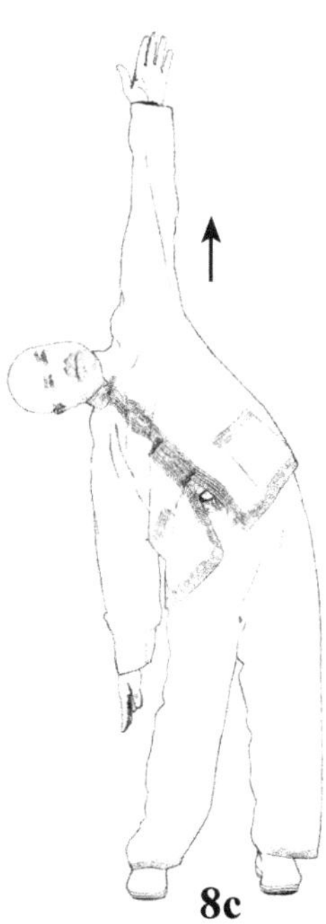

**8c**

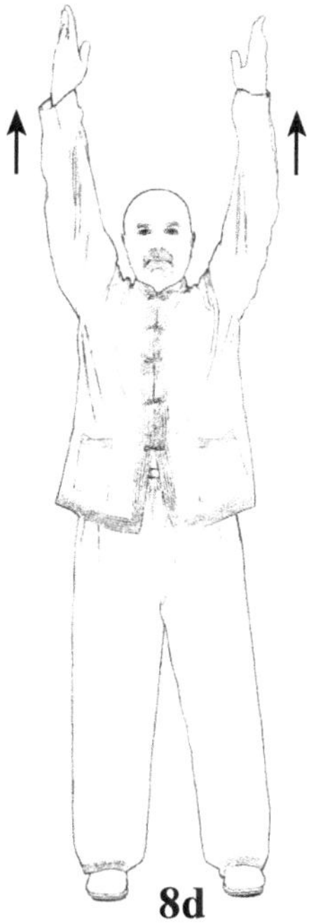

**8d**

**8c-d**  Raise your right arm up over your head and then raise your left arm. With the palms of your hands facing each other and fingers pointing to the sky stretch up, lifting your spine.

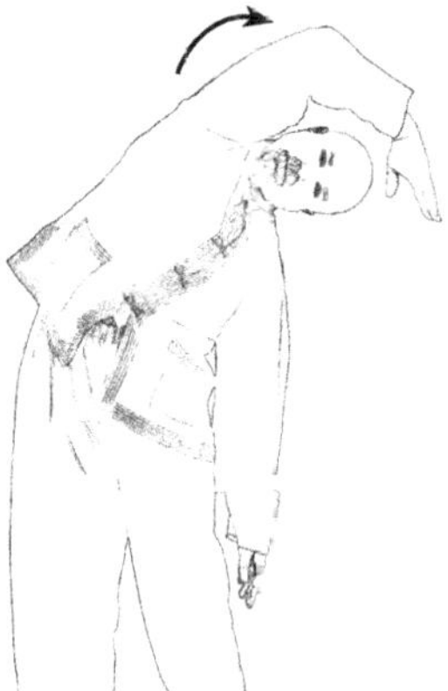

**8e**

**8e**  Lower your right arm to the side of your body and lean to your right with your left arm circling over your head; fingers are pointing towards the ground and your eyes are looking towards the sky. With each out breath stretch a little more. Continue for a total of four breaths.

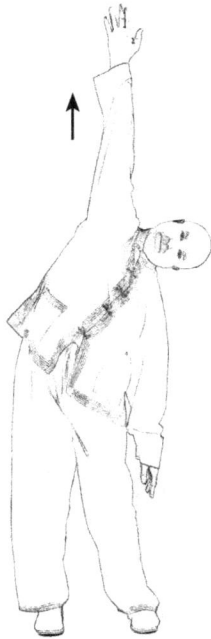

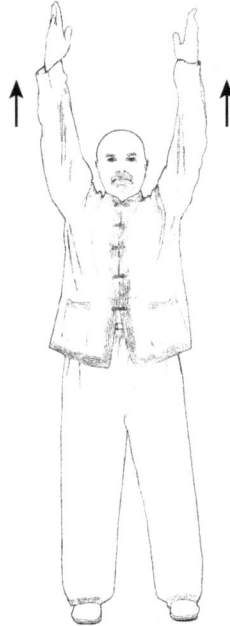

**8f**                                    **8g**

**8f-g**    Raise your left arm up over your head and then raise your right arm. With the palms of your hands facing each other and fingers pointing to the sky, stretch up, lifting your spine.

Repeat side stretch four times to each side.

# Front stretch

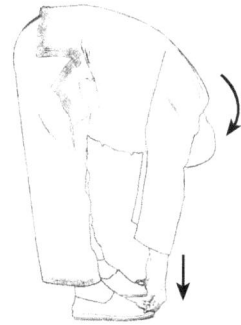

9a (side view)        9b (side view)        9c (side view)

**9a**    With your feet parallel and about shoulder-width apart, raise both arms up above your head. Pull the fingers of both hands back, pushing both palms up towards the sky. Stretch up, lifting your spine.

**9b**    Push your bottom back and lean forward, keeping your legs straight. With your fingers still pulled back, stretch forward, pushing both palms out and stretching your spine.

**9c**    Bend from your waist and fold in half. Keeping your legs straight allow your arms to naturally hang in front of your body with the knuckles of your hands resting on your feet. With each out breath stretch a little more. Continue for a total of four breaths.

**9d (side view)**        **9e (side view)**        **9f (side view)**

**9d-f**   Gently bend your knees and slowly straighten your back, lifting your upper body from the waist. Keep your shoulders and neck relaxed, and the chin on your chest. Your eyes are looking at the ground. It is important to raise the neck and head last, after the body is upright.

Repeat front stretch four times.

# Body roll

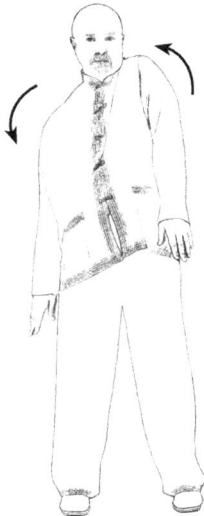

**10a** **10b**

**10a-b**  Let your arms slowly descend to your sides. Slowly roll one shoulder and then the other, like swimming backstroke. With your awareness, feel the motion massage your shoulders, chest, your abdomen, and your back over the kidney area.

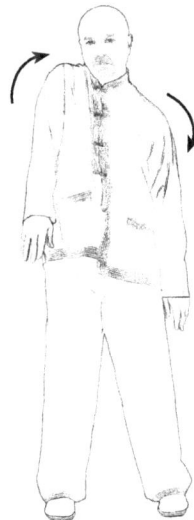

**10c** **10d**

**10c-d**  After about 8 rotations, stop and come back the other way, rotating forward, and feel the internal massage.

## Body swings

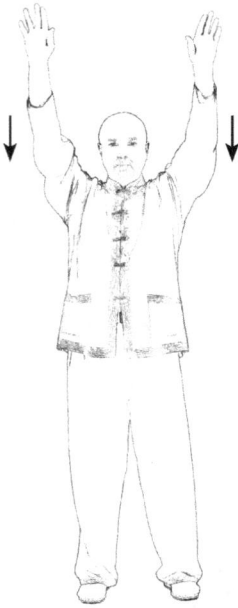 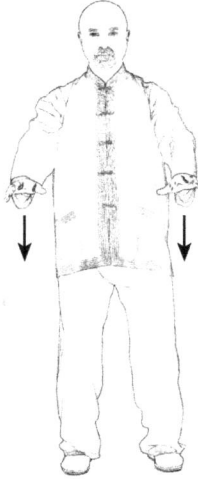 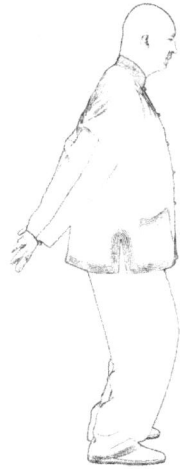

**11a**             **11b**             **11c (side view)**

**11a-c** With the feet parallel and arms above the head, swing the arms down, sinking the knees at the same time. Let the whole body swing; keep the back straight and head upright. With your awareness, relax the shoulders and hips, elbows and knees, wrists and ankles, hands and feet. Do this for about 12 swings. This helps strengthen the whole body and is good for blood circulation.

# Swinging arms

**12a-c** Step out to a wider horse-riding stance. With the legs grounded firmly and the arms relaxed, let your arms swing out, turning from the waist. Let the arms slap across the body, massaging around the waist and hips.

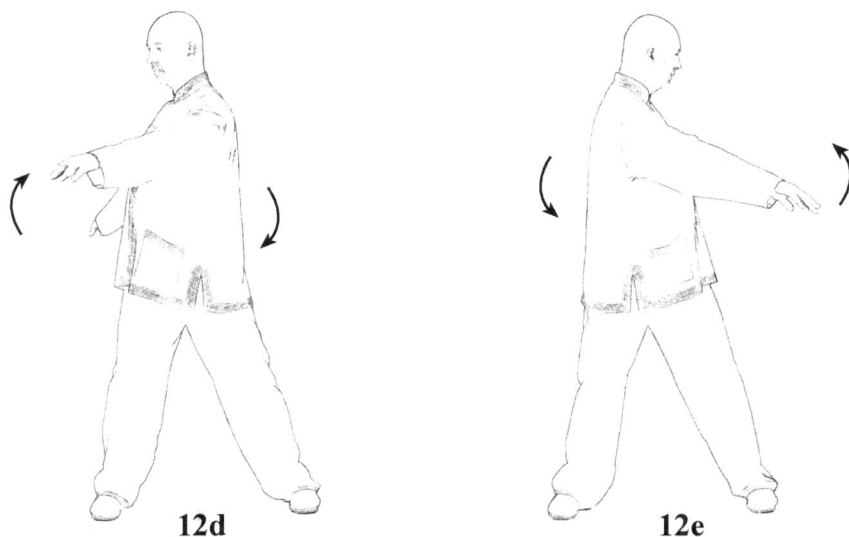

**12d-e** Let your arms swing higher, massaging around the kidneys and finally, higher again as one swinging arm taps the shoulder while the other taps the kidneys. Do this 12 times.

This helps loosen and strengthen the back and massage the internal organs.

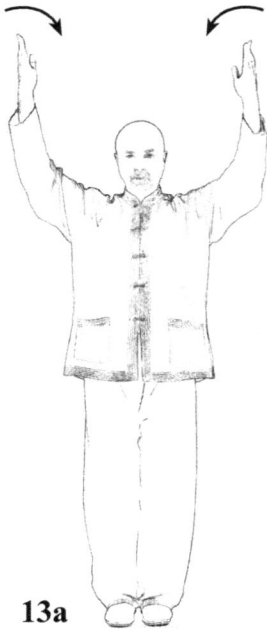

**13a**                               **13b**

**13a-b** Stand with your feet together; raise your hands up above your head guiding the Qi down the body from the top of the head to the soles of your feet. Your arms rest naturally at the side of your body. With your eyes closed, relax from the top of your head down to your hands and down to your feet; relax down through the body on the out breath. Stay in this position and allow the Qi to settle for a few minutes.

**13c**                               **13d**

**13c-d** With your eyes closed, relax from the top of your head down to your hands and down to your feet; relax down through the body on the out breath. Stay in this position and allow the Qi to settle for a few minutes.

**We are now ready to practise our Qigong.**

# Chapter 6
# The 2nd 64 Movements

Da Yan - Wild Goose Qigong
The 2nd 64 movements

# Da Yan – Wild Goose Qigong
# The 2nd 64 Movements
# 大雁气功后64式

The 2nd 64 movement Dayan Wild Goose Qigong continues on from where the 1st 64 movement set finished.

Practising the 2nd 64 movement set on its own
When practising the 2nd 64 movement set on its own, begin with the same opening movements as the 1st 64 movement set.

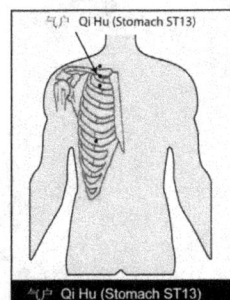

Qi Hu (Stomach ST13)

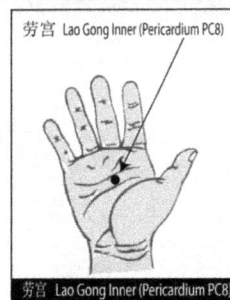

Qi Hu (Stomach ST13)

劳宫 Lao Gong Inner (Pericardium PC8)

劳宫 Lao Gong Inner (Pericardium PC8)

a                                    b

Facing the Western direction:

**a** With your eyes gently closed, stand upright; the jaw is relaxed with the tip of the tongue placed gently on the roof of the mouth, just beneath the front teeth. Breathe naturally in and out through the nose. Your shoulders are relaxed, arms rounded and palms facing the body. The hands are relaxed with fingers open and slightly curled. The legs are straight with knees slightly off lock and with feet together. With your awareness and breath, relax from the top of your head to the soles of your feet; relax down through the body on the out breath.

Open your eyes and with your awareness focus out to the distance (looking, but not looking). Stay in this position for at least 30 seconds regulating mind, body and breath.

环跳 Huan Tiao (Gallbladder GB30)

环跳 Huan Tiao (Gallbladder GB30)

涌泉 Yong Quan (Kidney K1)

涌泉 Yong Quan (Kidney K1)

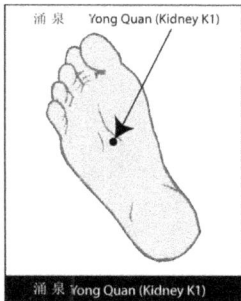

**b** Lower the knees and sink down moving your bodyweight slightly to the right. Stepping to the left with the left foot making a small semi-circle on the ground, evenly distribute your weight with your feet no wider than shoulder-width apart.

Open your chest slightly with arms rounded away from the body, stimulating the Qi Hu (Stomach ST13) located just below the middle of the collar bone. The Lao Gong (Pericardium PC8) in the middle of the palm faces towards the Huan Tiao (Gallbladder GB30) point at the hip joint at the indentation on either side of the buttocks.

Standing in this position allows the Qi to flow through the whole body, from head to feet. Connecting the Lao Gong (middle of palm) with the Huan Tiao (hip) stimulates the Qi down the Gall Bladder Channel and by opening the chest this helps stimulate the Qi Hu (beneath collar bone), allowing the Qi to move down to the Huan Tiao (hip) and down to the Yong Quan (Kidney K1) at the soles of the feet.

**Practising both sets of 64 together**
When practising both sets together, finish the first set with the following closing movement:

**b** The arms circle around the body and the hands scan around the waist until the Lao Gong (middle of palm) faces the Huan Tiao (Gallbladder GB30) point at the hip joint which is at the indentation on either side of the buttocks.

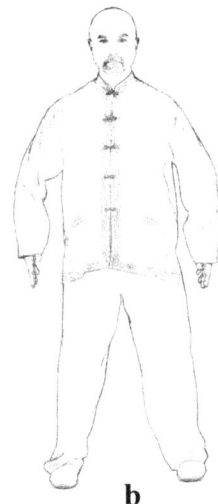

b

# 1. Sleeping peacefully 安睡

*This first movement has the same benefits as the closing movement of the 1st 64 movement set. It brings the refined Qi to the Lower Dan Tian (beneath the navel) and stimulates the Heavenly Orbit.*

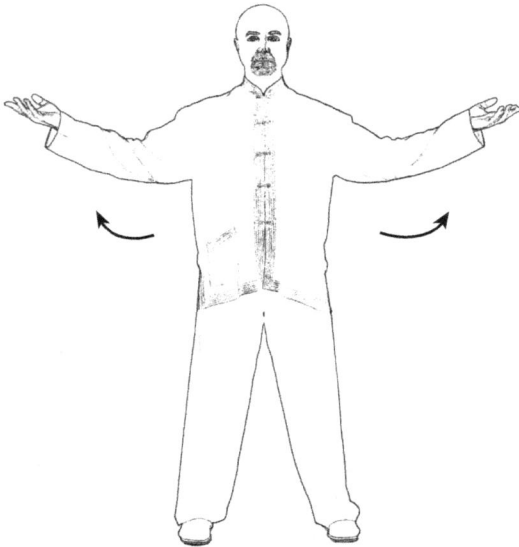 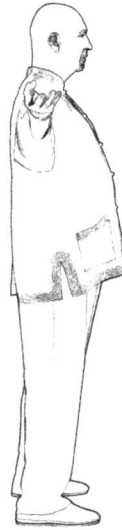 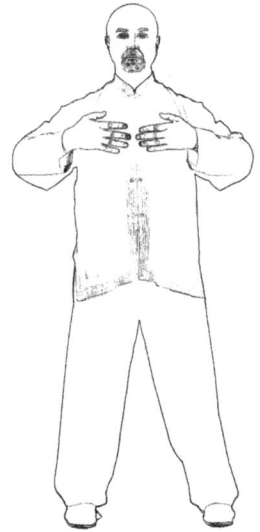

**1a**  **1a side view**  **1b**

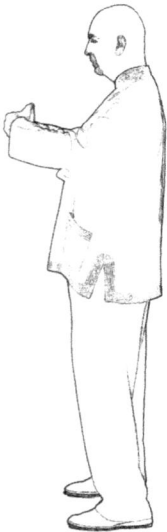 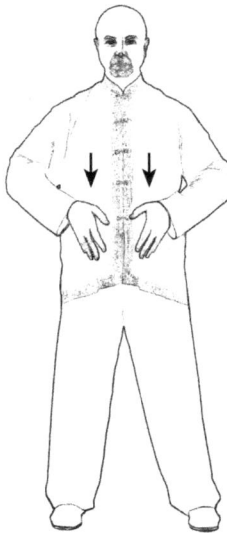

**1b side view**  **1c**

**1a** Rotate the wrists whilst arms are down by the side so the palms are facing up to the sky. Raise your arms to the side to shoulder height keeping shoulders, elbows and hands relaxed and soft.

**1b** With the palms facing the sky absorbing the heaven Qi move both arms toward the front of the body. Turn the palms to face the chest, bringing a big ball of Qi into the heart. The elbows are relaxed, fingers are facing each other and the palms point towards the chest.

**1c** Move your hands down in front of the body with the fingers pointing to the Lower Dan Tian (area beneath the navel).

**1d**                          **1d side view**

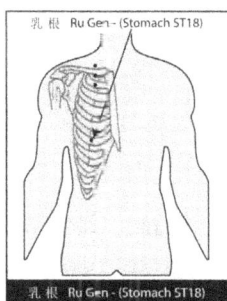

**1d** The middle fingers touch the Dai Mai (Gall Bladder GB26) at the side of the body below the 11th rib at the same height as the navel with thumbs on Ru Gen (Stomach ST18) beneath the middle of the ribs which is the 5th intercostal space just below the nipple. Squat down with your bodyweight over the balls of the feet, lifting both heels off the ground. Both palms sit around the abdominal area. Allow Qi to settle at the Lower Dan Tian (area beneath the navel). This is the same as the finishing position in the 1st 64 movement set but you only stay in this position for a few seconds.

**Benefit:** This movement improves cardiovascular health and arthritis.

## 2. Stretching the claw 伸爪

*This movement creates a Qi field around the whole body by stimulating the energy Channels from the head to the toes.*

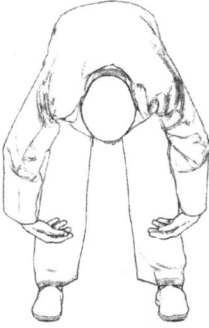 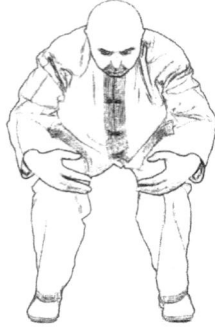 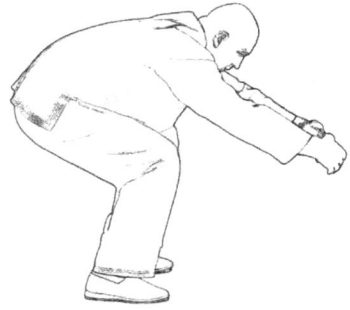

2a                 2b              2b side view

**2a** Slightly straighten your legs and place your heels on the ground. The hands move down and scan the inside of your legs with the back of your hands.

**2b** Bend the legs again and whilst in this position move the arms up with the fingers facing each other as if holding a large ball in the arms. Gently lift the upper body from the waist to an angle of about 45°.

**Benefit:** This movement improves digestion and Bladder and Kidney function.

# 3. Withdrawing the arms 收膀

*In this movement the flow of Qi is strengthened into the three Channels –*
*Spleen, Kidney and Gall Bladder – nurturing Kidney yang energy.*

3a

3b

京 门 Jing Men (Gall Bladder GB25)

京 门 Jing Men (Gall Bladder GB25)

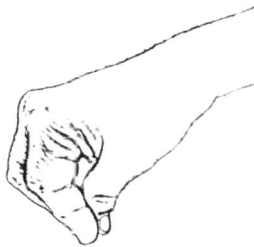

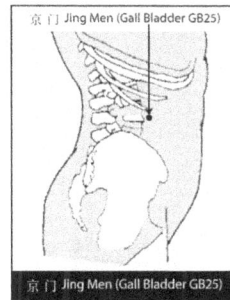

**3a** Move your bodyweight to the right and pivot on the left heel turning the body 90° to face the Southern direction. Maintain the waist at an angle of about 45°. At the same time, relax the wrists and turn both palms to the left, sweeping the arms around in coordination with the body.

**3b** The left hand circles in towards the body, scooping in the Qi and forming a Plum Blossom Claw (four fingers touching together with the thumb) which is turned upward and touching the Jing Men (Gall Bladder GB25) at the side of the body at the free end of the 12 rib. The right palm turns in toward the face and centre of the chest. Eyes are looking at the right hand. Your bodyweight is on the right leg with the left heel lifted slightly and about 60% pressure on the front of the foot.

3c

3d

3e

**3c** Turn your body 180° to face the Northern direction. Pivoting on the left heel, hook in the left toe as far as feels comfortable. At the same time, relax the left wrist and release the left Plum Blossom Claw (four fingers touching together with the thumb) with the palm turning to the right and the body moving in a clockwise direction.

**3d** Move your bodyweight back over the left leg and pivot on the right heel turning the toes to face the Northern direction. Maintain the waist at an angle of about 45°.

**3e** The right hand circles in towards the body, scooping in the Qi and forming a Plum Blossom Claw (four fingers touching together with the thumb) which is turned upward and touching the Jing Men (bottom of ribs). The left palm turns in toward the face and centre of the chest. Eyes are looking at the left hand. Your bodyweight is on the left leg with the right heel lifted slightly and about 60% pressure on the front of the foot.

**Benefit:** These movements help stimulate the Kidneys, digestive system and can improve the complexion. They also relieve tension in the back and waist.

# 4. Sighting the wind 寻风

*This movement creates an energy field by holding the arms in a circular position in front of the body which stimulates the Middle Dan Tian (middle of chest between the nipples).*

4a                                      4b                                      4c

**4a** With your bodyweight still on the left leg, relax your right wrist and release the right Plum Blossom Claw (four fingers touching together with the thumb). Lift your right arm, with fingers of each hand now facing each other and the palms facing your chest. Keep both elbows relaxed as if holding a large ball on the chest. At the same time, gently straighten your back and lift the upper body from the waist, keeping your shoulders and chest relaxed. When the arms come up the foot comes up; your knees remain bent, your right toes are pointing upward and the eyes are looking straight ahead.

**4b** Pivot on your right heel turning the right toe and your body 90° to face the Western direction. Straighten your legs slightly and stand a little taller.

**4c** Lower the knees slightly and move your bodyweight over the right leg pivoting on the left heel to turn the left toe 90°. Turn the whole body to face the Southern direction.

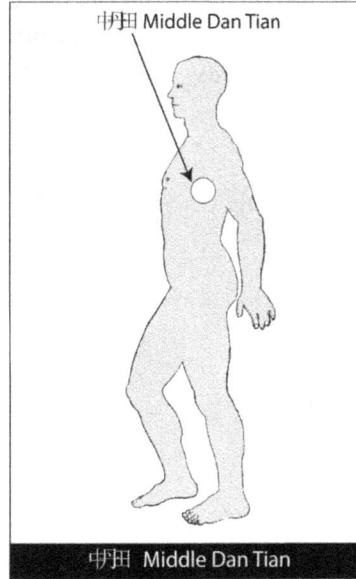

中丹田 Middle Dan Tian

中丹田 Middle Dan Tian

**4d**

**4d** Maintain your bodyweight over the right leg and pivot on the left heel turning your left toe and whole body 90° to face the Western direction.

**Benefit:** This movement improves brain function and the posture of the upper body.

## 5.   Pulling the claws back to the shoulders 背抓对肩

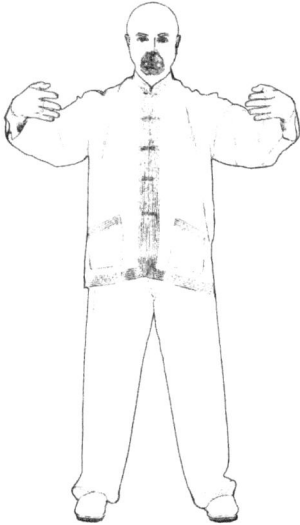 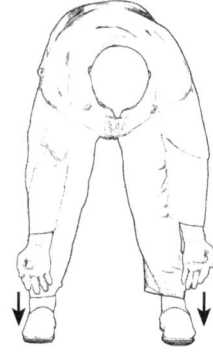

5a                5b                5c

**5a**      With a soft hand and the thumb relaxed (imagine holding an egg), slowly separate the arms with the fingers still facing each other, being aware of the Qi between the fingers.

**5b**      Relax the shoulders and move both arms to the side of the body. Gently push the bottom back as you stretch forward and bend from the waist.

**5c**      The hands, with palms turned up to face the sky, slowly scan down the outside of both legs to the feet.

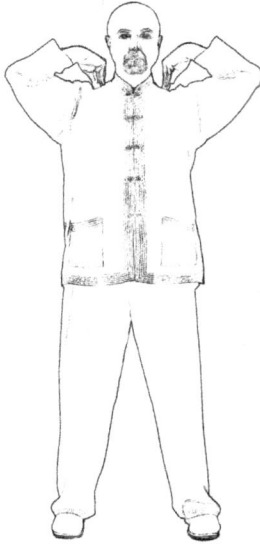

5d      5d side view

**5d**      Gently bend the knees and lift the upper body from the waist, keeping your shoulders and chest relaxed. The arms rise up with the body to over the head. Forming the Plum Blossom Claw (four fingers touching together with the thumb) on both hands, touch the Jian Jing (Gall Bladder GB21) which the highest point between the shoulder and the neck.

**Benefit:** This movement joins the points of three different Channels – Gall Bladder, Stomach and Triple Burner. It releases dampness (phlegm) and is good for headaches, shoulder problems and the common cold.

## 6.    Dispelling the bad Qi 散病气

*In this movement congested Qi is thrown away from the Liver, Stomach and Spleen, and helps regulate the digestive system.*

| | | |
|---|---|---|
| **6a** | **6b** | **6c** |

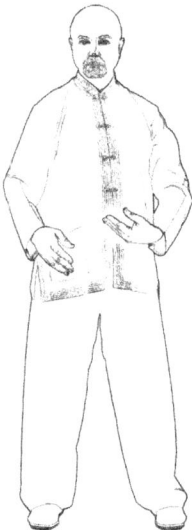

**6d**

**6a,b**    Keep your bodyweight centred and look straight ahead. Release both Plum Blossom Claws (four fingers touching together with the thumb). The right hand moves down past the Qi Hu (beneath collar bone) to the abdomen and quickly flicks out in front of the body. The palm is facing the ground dispelling the bad Qi to the earth.

**6c,d**    Repeat the same movement with the left hand. Finish the movement with the left hand closer to the body.

# 7.    Rotating the hands 缠手

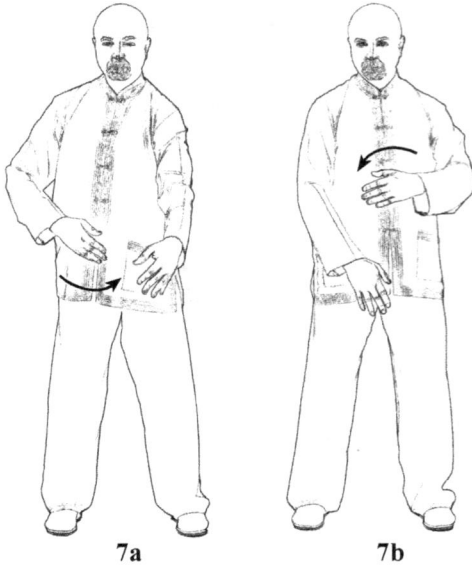

7a

7b

**7a**    Keep your bodyweight centred and look straight ahead. Rotate the right hand towards the body with the right hand moving up under the left hand.

**7b**    Rotate one complete circle with the hands about 5cm apart finishing with the left hand closest to the body.

**Benefit:** This movement improves the digestive system, strengthens the cardiovascular system, and stimulates the Triple Burner, Liver and Gall Bladder Channels.

## Step right

**7c**    Rotate hands half a circle and at the same time step forward by bringing your bodyweight over the left leg and gently placing the outer part of the right foot (small toe) half a step in front, only just touching. Eyes are looking straight ahead. The rotating of the hands finishes with the left hand closest to the body.

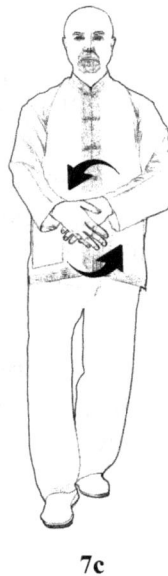

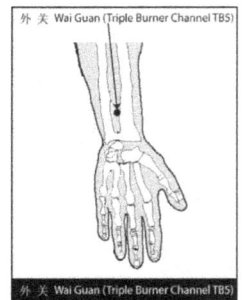

7c

内关 Nei Guan (Pericardium Channel PC6)

内关 Nei Guan (Pericardium Channel PC6)

外关 Wai Guan (Triple Burner Channel TB5)

外关 Wai Guan (Triple Burner Channel TB5)

## Step left

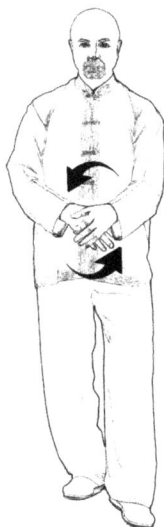

7d

**7d** Rotate hands half a circle and at the same time step forward and bring your bodyweight over the right leg and gently place the outer part of the left foot (small toe) half a step in front only just touching. Eyes are looking straight ahead. The rotating of the hands finishes with the right hand closest to the body.

## Step right

**7e** Rotate hands half a circle and at the same time step forward by bringing your bodyweight over the left leg and gently place the outer part of the right foot (small toe) half a step in front, only just touching. Eyes are looking straight ahead. The rotating of the hands finishes with the left hand closest to the body.

In this movement you are rotating two points around each other, the Nei Guan (Pericardium Channel PC6) in the middle of the inner arm which is between the two bones about 5cm from the wrist, and the point directly opposite on the outer arm, the Wai Guan (Triple Burner Channel TB5) on the outside between the two bones about 5cm from the wrist. Look at the hands whilst rotating them.

7d

These stepping movements are similar to a Dayan or great bird gently stepping forward.

## 8.  Turning the body and sending back the Qi 转身收气

*These movements pump blood up to the head which brings Qi up the Du Channel into the head and brain.*

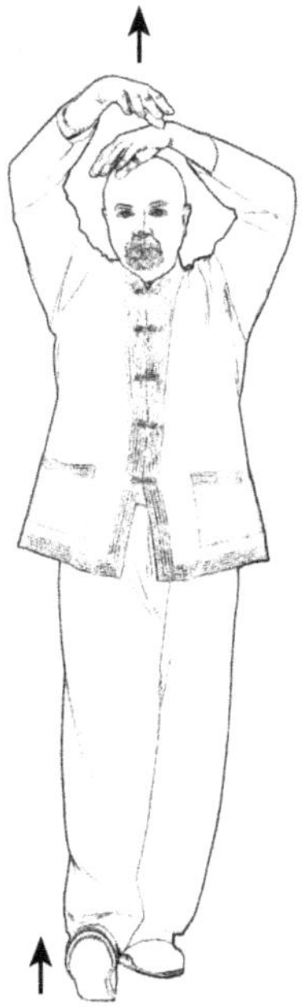

**8a side view** 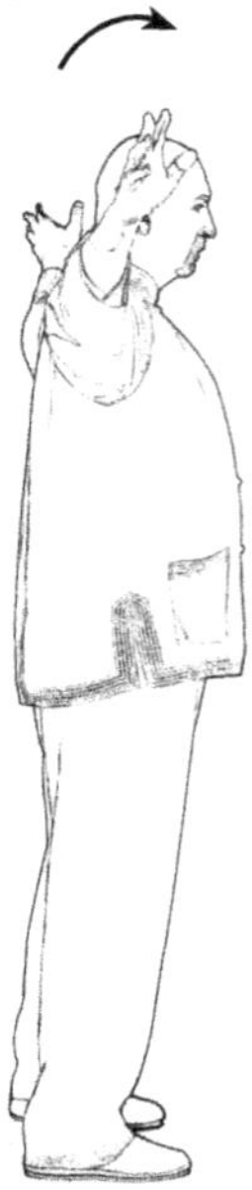      **8b** 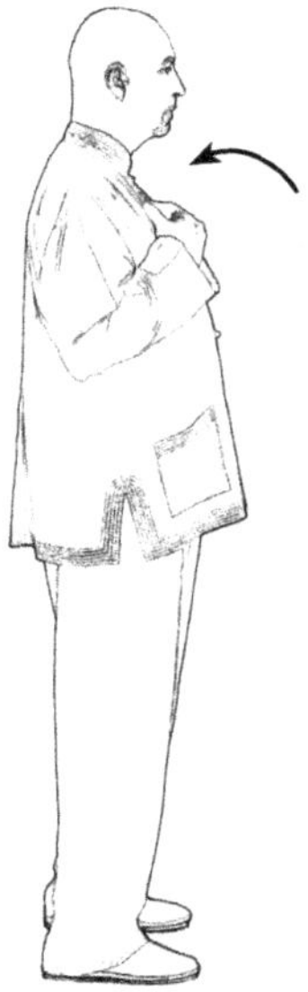      **8c** 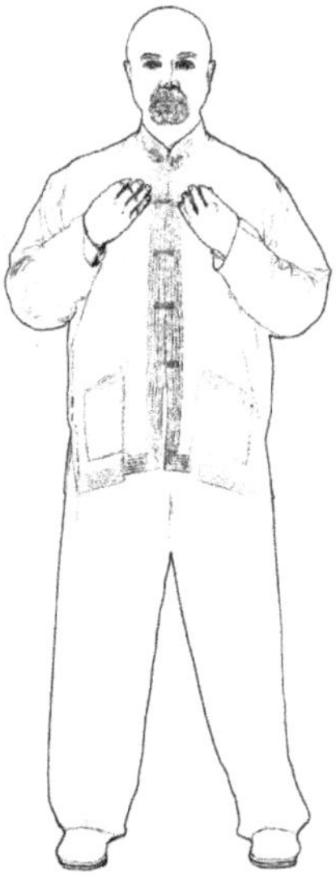      **8c side view**

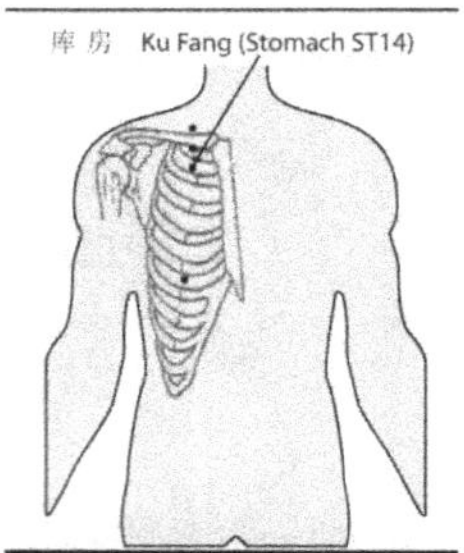

库房  Ku Fang (Stomach ST14)

库房  Ku Fang (Stomach ST14)

**8a,b**   Lift the right toes off the ground, pivot on the right heel turning the right toes 90°. At the same time pivot on the left foot and turn the whole body to face the Southern direction. The arms lift with the body, keeping shoulders and elbows relaxed.

**8c**   The arms circle down to the side of the body and the hands move up in front of your chest. The Lao Gong (middle of palm) of both hands are facing both Ku Fang (Stomach ST14) between the collar bone and the nipple.

**8d** Keep the feet parallel, the knees straight and your bodyweight evenly distributed. Facing the Southern direction, turn the upper body from the waist slowly sweeping 180° to the right to face the Northern direction.

**8e** Then turning from the waist slowly turn the upper body 360° with the eyes sweeping around the horizon to again face the Northern direction.

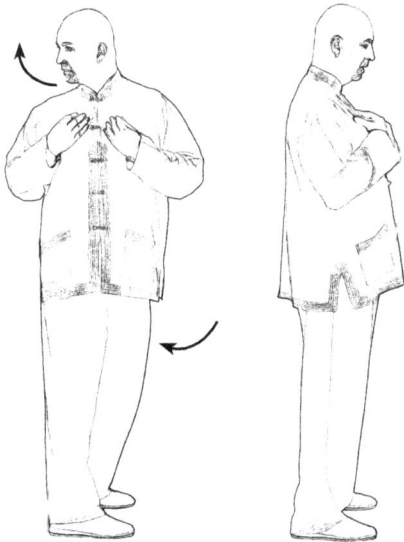

8d          8e

**8f** Repeat the 360° turn to the right facing the Northern direction.

**8g** Turn the body 180° to face the Southern direction.

**Benefit:** These movements improve the blood circulation of the Heart which increases Heart energy. It also increases brain function, improves blood circulation around the body and spinal nerve function, and helps with neck and shoulder problems.

8f          8g

# 9. Dispelling the bad Qi 甩病气

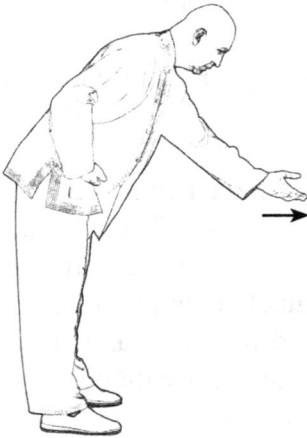

**9a**  Keep your feet parallel, the knees slightly bent and your bodyweight evenly distributed. Lower both arms with the fingers gently touching the skin, from the Qi Hu (beneath collar bone), down the Stomach Channel and to the Dai Mai (below the ribs).

**9b**  Softly flick the right hand out to dispel bad Qi; the fingers face the ground, the palm faces upwards and the body leans forward with the flicking movement.

**9c**  Slowly straighten the body as the right hand moves back with the palm face up and the fingers gently touching the Dai Mai (below the ribs).

**9d**  Repeat the movement with the left hand, softly flicking out to dispel the bad Qi; the body leans forward slightly with the fingers facing the ground and the palm upwards. Slowly straighten the body as the left hand moves back with the palm facing up and the fingers gently touching the Dai Mai (below the ribs).

**Benefit:** Dispelling of the bad (stale) Qi benefits the chest and Stomach.

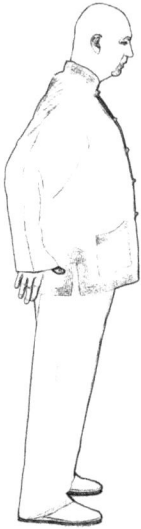
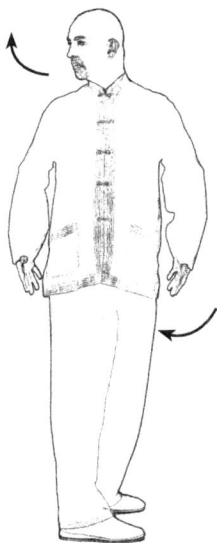

**9e,f** Lift both arms to about shoulder height, rotating the hands inward then away from the body; the palms are facing the front. Slightly straighten your elbows and gently push the hands out in front in line with the shoulders, keeping the shoulders relaxed. Pause to feel the Qi, about two to three seconds.

**9e**            **9f**

## 10. Bringing back the wings and holding the Qi 背翅抱气

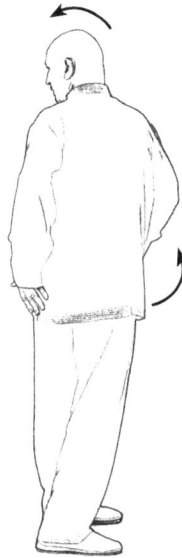

**10a** Circle both arms out and around behind the body to connect the Lao Gong (middle of palm) with the Huan Tiao (hip) at the indentation on either side of the buttocks. Keep the shoulders and elbows relaxed.

**10b** Keep the feet parallel, the knees straight and your bodyweight evenly distributed. Facing

**10a**            **10b**            **10c**

the Southern direction turn the upper body from the waist slowly sweeping around 180° to the right facing the Northern direction.

**10c** Then turning from the waist slowly turn the upper body 360° to the left with the eyes sweeping around the horizon to face the Northern direction.

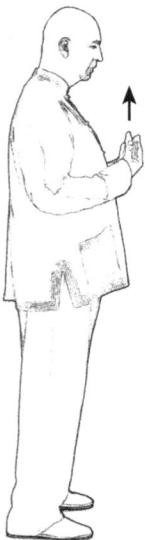

**10d** Repeat the 360° turn again to the right facing the Northern direction.

**10e** Turn the body 180° to face the Southern direction.

**Benefit:** This movement exercises and regulates muscles, tendons, joints and nerves and is good for blood pressure control.

**10d**          **10e**

## 11.  Distributing and moving away the Qi 贯气 排气

*As the hands pass over the head they receive Qi from the main acupressure points of the head. Bad Qi is then dispersed down through the Stomach Channel.*

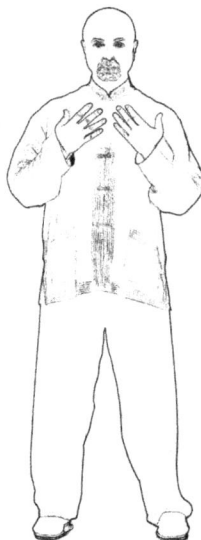

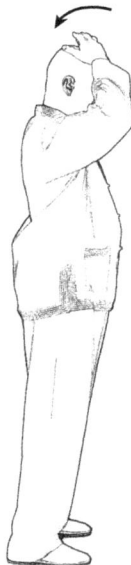

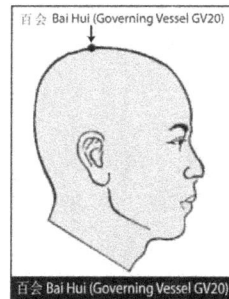

**11a**     **11a side view**     **11b**

**11a** Rotate both hands in towards the front of the body. Keeping shoulders and chest relaxed, scoop your hands up scanning the front of the body. Palms are facing towards the body and fingers are pointing up to the sky at a distance of about 3cm from the surface of the body.

**11b** Your hands pass over the face and move over the Bai Hui (top of the head) and continue scanning down the back of the head.

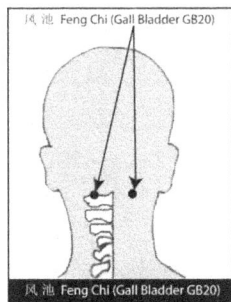

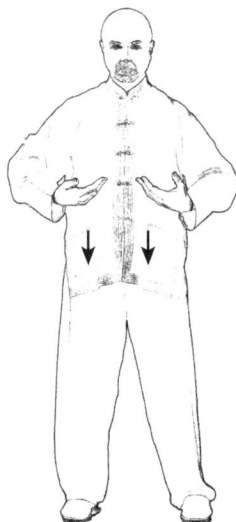

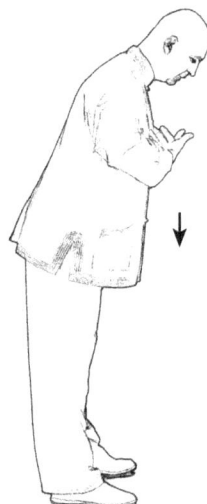

**11c**                    **11d side view**                    **11d**

**11c,d**  Keep your shoulders relaxed and rotate both hands so palms are facing the Feng Chi (Gall Bladder GB20) at the base of the scull. The hands continue moving down with the back of the fingers moving past the Qi Hu (beneath collar bone) and moving further down past the Dai Mai (below the ribs).

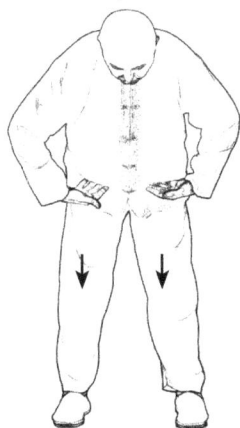

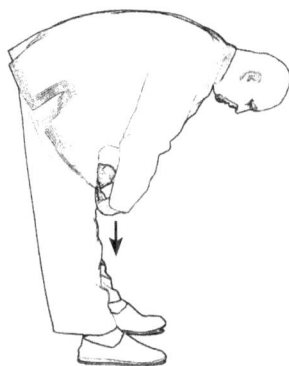

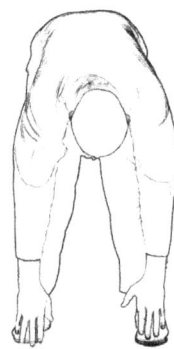

**11e side view**                    **11e**                    **11f side view**

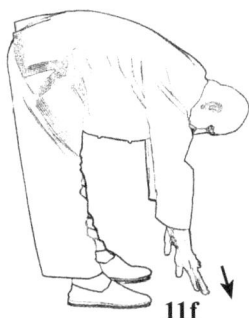

**11f**

**11e**   Keeping the legs straight, gently push the bottom back as you stretch forward and bend from the waist. Your hands continue to gently scan the inside of the legs.

**11f**   When the hands are over the feet, quickly flick them out making a flicking sound. The palms are facing the ground, dispelling the bad Qi.

## 12. Crossing the hands through the legs 穿叉

*This movement opens the Sanjiao (Triple Burner).*

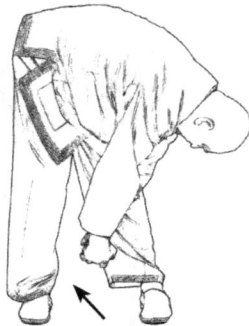 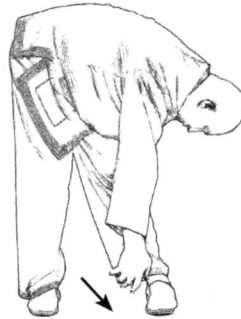 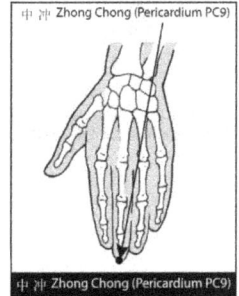

| 12a | 12a side view | 12b side view |

**12a**  Keeping the legs straight gently turn from the waist to the left, keeping your chest open and arms rounded. The left arm is behind the body and the right arm in front. Bring the Zhong Chong (Pericardium PC9), tip of the middle fingers on both hands together between the legs.

**12b**  Quickly separate the hands.

**Benefit:** Movements 12, 13 and 14 are good for leg and back problems including sciatica and the Bladder.

This movement improves brain function and is a strong, powerful movement that helps reduce menstrual pain and is good for the Large Intestine.

# 13.Distributing the Qi into the outer side of the ankles
外踝骨贯气

*This movement distributes Qi through the Kunlun belt area around the outside of the feet (Bladder Channel).*

**Right ankle**

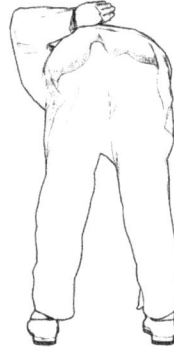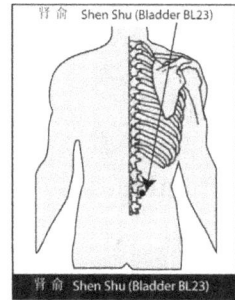

13a            13a side view     13a side (back) view

**13a** Keeping the legs straight and bent over from the waist turn the body to face the Southern direction. Bring the left arm to the back so the He Gu (web of hand) is touching the Shen Shu (Bladder BL23) behind the navel, either side of the spine beneath the Kidneys. The right Lao Gong (middle of palm) is facing the Jie Xi (Stomach ST41) at the front in the centre of the ankle

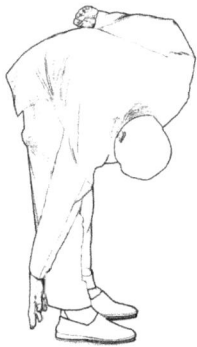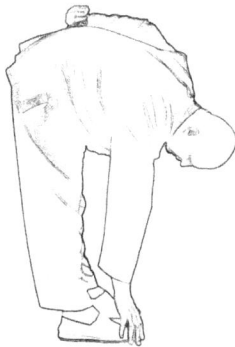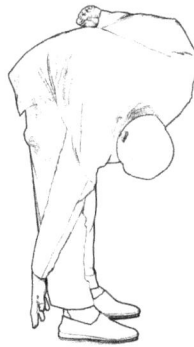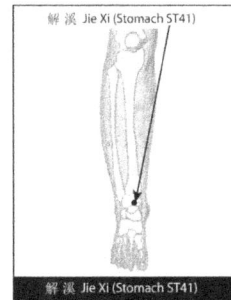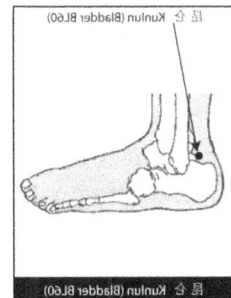

← 13b          → 13c          ←13d

**13b,c,d** Turning from the waist, the right Lao Gong (middle of palm) scans around the outside of the right ankle distributing the Qi to the Kunlun (Bladder BL60), the depression above the heel, and then back to the front and then back to the heel again. The eyes are looking at the hand.          Repeat three times

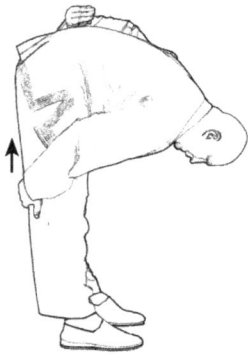

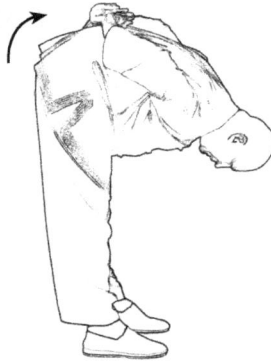

**13e,f** Lift your right arm to the back so the He Gu (web of hand) is touching the Shen Shu (beneath Kidneys).

13e        13f

**Left ankle**

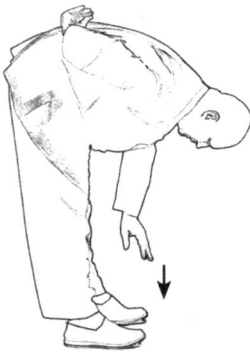

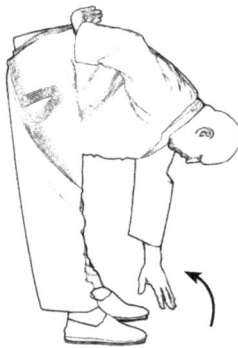

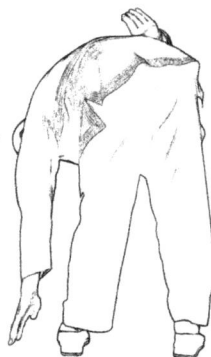

13g     13h     13h side (back view)   13i side (back view)

**13g** Lower your left arm with the palm facing the foot. The left Lao Gong (middle of palm) is facing the Jie Xi (front of ankle).

**13h,i** Turning from the waist the left Lao Gong (middle of palm) scans around the outside of the left ankle distributing the Qi to the Kunlun (depression behind ankle) and then back to the front and then back to the heel again. The eyes are looking at the hand.        Repeat three times

**Benefit:** This set of movements ease stress and is good for head, neck and shoulder problems. This is a slow, soft and smooth movement. As your flexibility increases try to make the movement precise for better benefits. Precise movement and the energy connections are the foundations for advanced practice.

# 14. Rubbing the legs 搓背，搓腿

*The hands soothe the Bladder Channel by gently rubbing the back of the legs.*

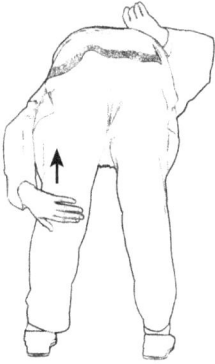

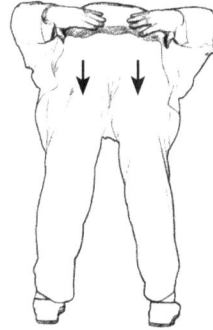

14a side (back) view            14b            14c side (back) view

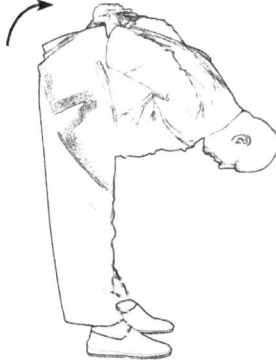

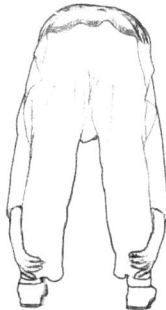

**14a** Lift the left arm up the back of the leg and continue up the back so the He Gu (web of hand) is touching the Shen Shu (beneath Kidneys).

**14b** Raise both hands up the back along the Bladder Channel as far as feels comfortable.

**14c** Turn hands over so both palms are touching the mid-back area.

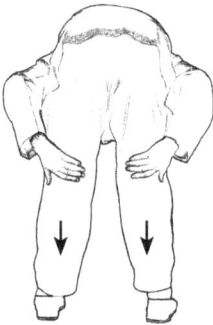

14d side (back) view       14e side (back) view            14e

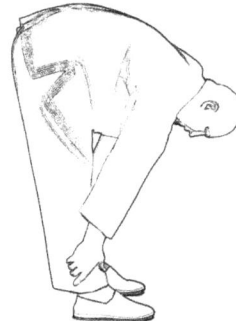

**14d,e** Move your hands down the back rubbing over the backside, down the outside of the legs to the lower part of the calves.

## 15. Clap the hands 拍掌

*Clapping the hands vibrates Qi to the 3rd eye. This follows the Heart Channel. It stimulates the five organs, mainly providing Qi to support the Heart*

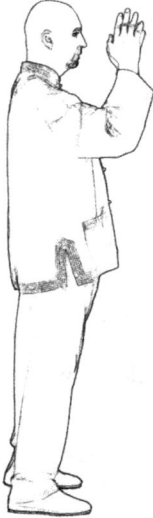

15a

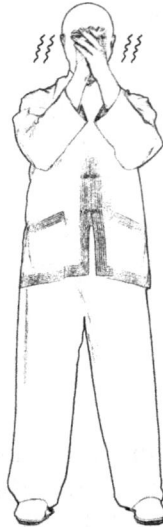

15a side view

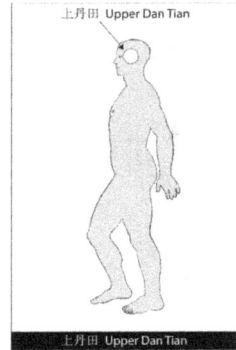

**15a** Gently bend your knees and lift the upper body from the waist, keeping the shoulders and chest relaxed. Your bodyweight is evenly distributed with the knees slightly bent. The arms rise with the body at a distance of about shoulder-width apart. Both hands clap softly in front of the Upper Dan Tian, the area between the eyebrows. The eyes look at the hands which are relaxed and slightly hollow.

# 16. Rubbing the arms 搓臂

*The slapping of the hands stimulates the five senses of the face and the three Yang Channels of the arms.*

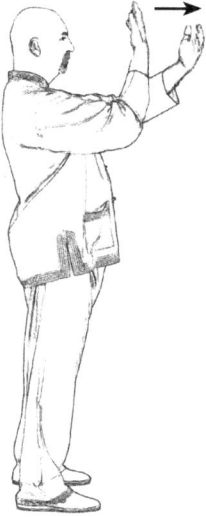

**16a** Turn both palms over to face the Upper Dan Tian (between the eyebrows). Keep your shoulders relaxed and elbows down.

**16b** Quickly slap the back of the right hand onto the palm of the left hand, looking at the palm.

16a    16b

## Rubbing the right arm

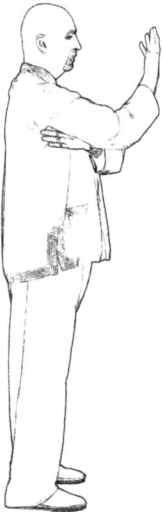
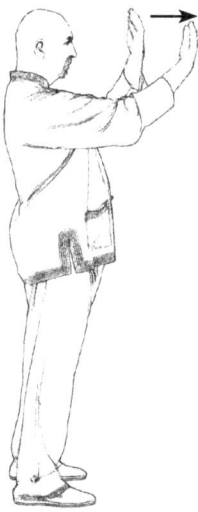
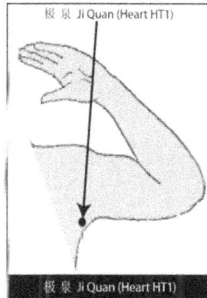

**16c** The left palm, with the Tiger's Mouth open (the thumb and index finger open to look like a tiger's mouth) wraps around the right arm and rubs down the outside of the arm stimulating the three Yang Channels (Small Intestine, Large Intestine and Triple Burner) and firmly slaps the Ji Quan (Heart HT1) under the right arm pit.

16c    16d

**16d** Move your left arm up in front of the body with left palm on the inside and both palms facing towards the Upper Dan Tian (between the eyebrows). Keep your shoulders relaxed and elbows down.

## Rubbing the left arm

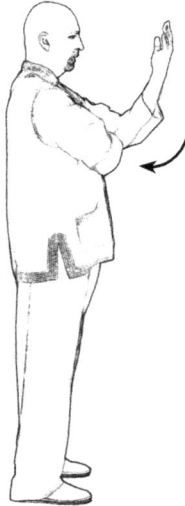

**16e** Quickly slap the back of the left hand onto the palm of the right hand, looking at the palm.

**16f** The right palm, with the Tiger's Mouth open, rubs down the outside of the left arm stimulating the three Yang Channels (Small Intestine, Large Intestine and Triple Burner) and firmly slaps the Ji Quan (Heart HT1) under the left arm pit.

16e          16f

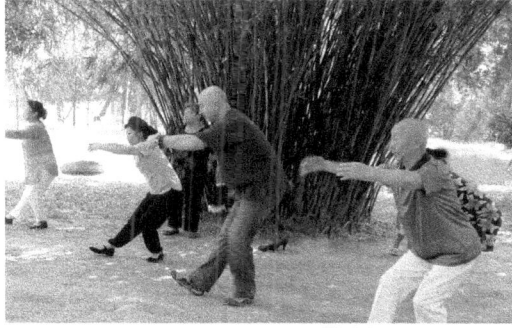

**Sighting the wind  寻 风**

**Bringing back the wings and holding the Qi 背 翅 抱 气**

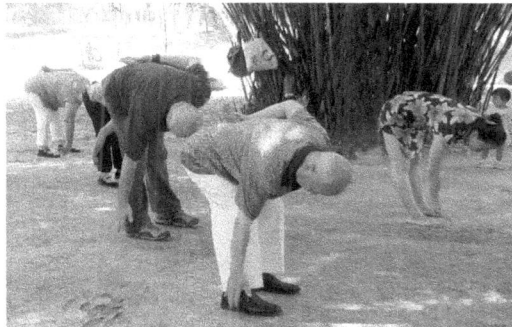

**Distributing the Qi into the outer side of the ankles 外 踝 骨 贯 气**

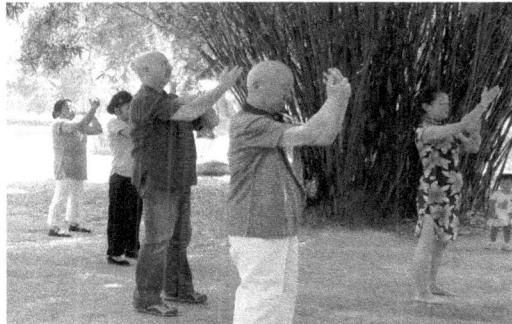

**Rubbing the arms 搓 臂**

# 17. Touching the points (seven touches) 点穴（七点）

*According to Traditional Chinese Medicine (TCM) the body is divided into three sections called the Sanjiao, which translates to the 'Triple Heater' or 'Burner'.*
*The Upper Heater relates to the organs above the diaphragm including the Thorax, Heart and Lungs, and aids the respiratory system of the body and heats up the air. The Upper Heater helps maintain the ability to absorb essence from the air and the universe.*

*The Middle Heater, located between the diaphragm and the navel, relates to the upper abdomen, the Spleen, Pancreas, Stomach, Liver, Gall Bladder and the Small Intestine. The Middle Heater functions like the oven of the body, heating the liquids and solids, and aiding in their digestion. The Middle*

*Heater promotes the absorption of essence from foods.*
*The Lower Heater, below the navel, relates to the organs of the lower abdomen including the Kidneys, Bladder and Large Intestine, and assists the elimination system of the body, also by heating up the solids and fluids.*

*The seven touches stimulate the major energy points allowing the Qi to flow smoothly through the Sanjiao.*

**Plum Blossom Claw:** The five fingers represent the five petals of the plum blossom and when all the fingers are joined, the five elements are united and together they stimulate the five major organs. This is used in many traditional practices within the martial arts and healing Qigong to direct Qi to a specific area

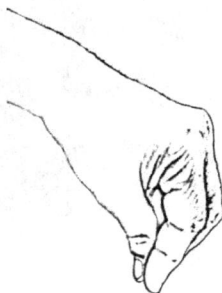

# First two touches for the Upper Heater

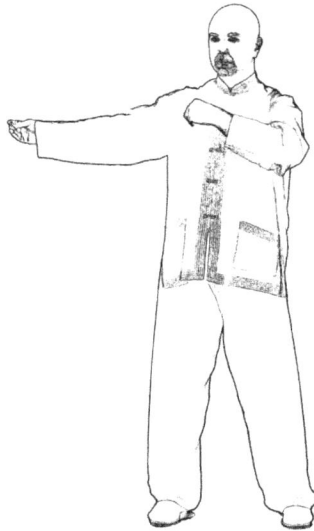

**17a side view**    **17b side view**

**17a,b** The feet are parallel and no wider than shoulder-width apart. Your bodyweight is evenly distributed and the knees slightly bent. Gently turning from the waist, swing the right arm so that the five fingers of the Plum Blossom Claw (four fingers touching together with the thumb) touch the left Qi Hu (beneath collar bone). Then, turning from the waist, swing the left arm so that the five fingers of the Plum Blossom Claw touch the right Qi Hu. At the same time, release the opposite Plum Blossom Claw and let the arm naturally swing out to the side.

**Benefit:** This movement aids the respiratory system and stimulates the Stomach Channel. It is good for relieving Stomach-ache.

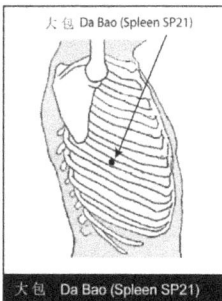

## Second two touches for the Middle Heater

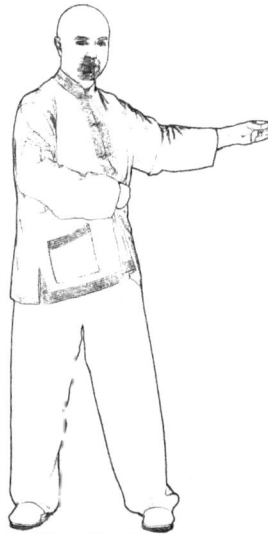

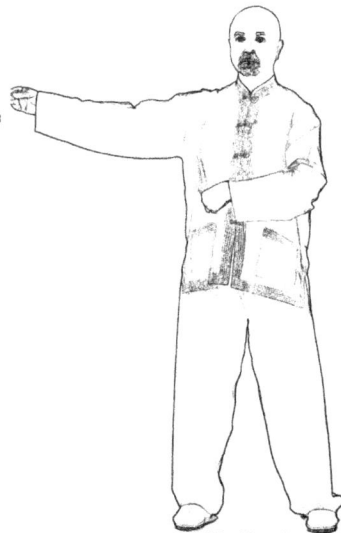

**17c,d** Gently turning from the waist, swing the right arm so that the five fingers of the Plum Blossom Claw touch the left Da Bao (Spleen SP21), the middle of the ribs at the side of the body. Then, turning from the waist, swing the left arm so that the five fingers of the Plum Blossom touch the right Da Bao.

**17c side view**    **17d side view**

**Benefit:** This movement stimulates the Spleen Channel and aids digestion.

## Third two touches for the Lower Heater

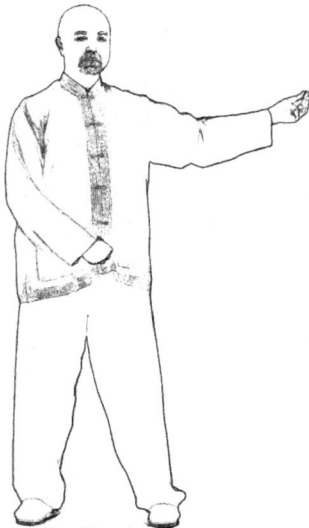

17e side view

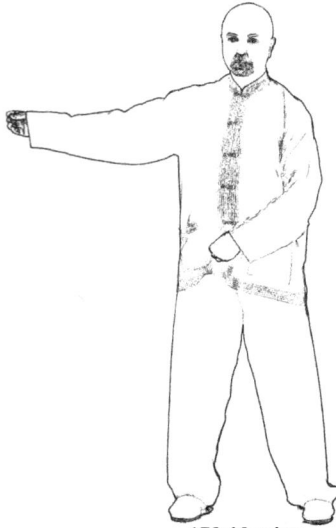

17f side view

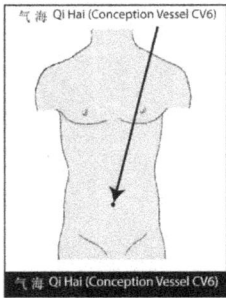

带脉 Dai Mai (Gall Bladder GB26)

带脉 Dai Mai (Gall Bladder GB26)

**17e,f** Swing the right arm turning from the waist so that the five fingers of the Plum Blossom Claw touch the left Dai Mai (below the ribs). Then, turning from the waist, swing the left arm so that the five fingers of the Plum Blossom Claw touch the Dai Mai on the opposite side. At the same time, release the opposite Plum Blossom Claw and let the arm naturally swing out to the side.

**Benefit:** This movement is good for the Gall Bladder and for relieving menstrual pain in women

### Seventh touch

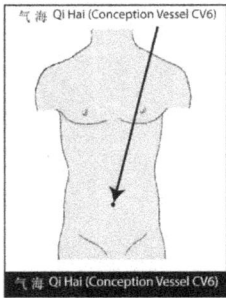

气海 Qi Hai (Conception Vessel CV6)

气海 Qi Hai (Conception Vessel CV6)

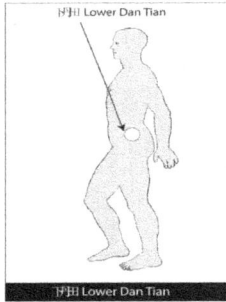

丹田 Lower Dan Tian

丹田 Lower Dan Tian

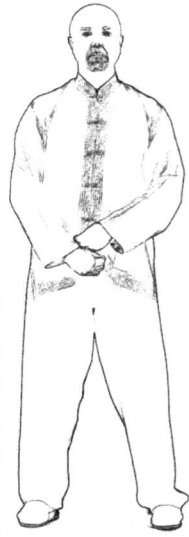

17g side view

17g  With the left Plum Blossom Claw remaining on the right Dai Mai (below the ribs), swing the right arm turning from the waist so that the five fingers of the Plum Blossom Claw touches the Qi Hai (Conception Vessel CV6) just beneath the navel allowing all the Qi to connect with the Lower Dan Tian (area beneath the navel).

**Benefit:** This movement stimulates the Lower Dan Tian (area beneath the navel), nurturing the Kidneys to reinforce original Qi. It also aids digestion and helps the five organs (Heart, Spleen, Lungs, Kidney and Liver) to function better.

## 18. Gathering the Qi 归气

*As described by Madam Chen, gathering the Qi is like 'gathering the peanuts'. It is important to pause at the end of this movement as it helps support original Qi*

18a side view            18b

**18a** The feet are parallel, no wider than shoulder-width apart. Your bodyweight is evenly distributed and the knees are slightly bent.

**18b** Relax the arms and circle the hands in towards the body. The palms face the lower abdomen. Stay in this position for about three seconds allowing Qi to settle at the Lower Dan Tian (area beneath the navel).

# 19. Crossing the arms 十字臂

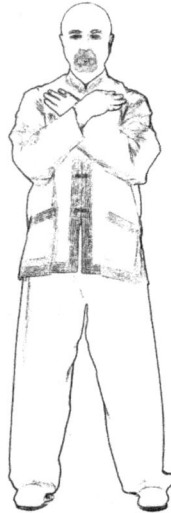

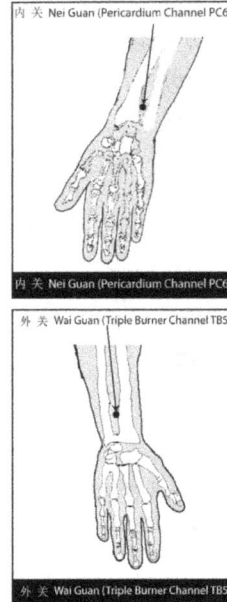

内 关 Nei Guan (Pericardium Channel PC6)

内 关 Nei Guan (Pericardium Channel PC6)

外 关 Wai Guan (Triple Burner Channel TB5)

外 关 Wai Guan (Triple Burner Channel TB5)

**19a side view**          **19b side view**

**19a** The feet and legs stay in the same position with the body facing the Southern direction. Both arms rise up in front of your body and cross at the wrist. The left arm is closer to the body. This connects two points: the Nei Guan (Pericardium Channel PC6) on the right arm which is in the middle of the inner edge of the arm between the two bones about 5cm from the wrist, and the point directly opposite on the outer edge of the left arm Wai Guan (Triple Burner Channel TB5) between the two bones about 5cm from the wrist.

**19b** The left Lao Gong (middle of palm) are gently placed over the right Ku Fang (between the collar bone and the nipple). The right Lao Gong is gently placed over the left Ku Fang. The eyes are looking straight ahead.

**Benefit:** This movement strengthens the Heart.

# 20. Sending down the Qi 下沉

*Sending down the Qi disperses the negative Qi to the ground through the soles of the feet.*

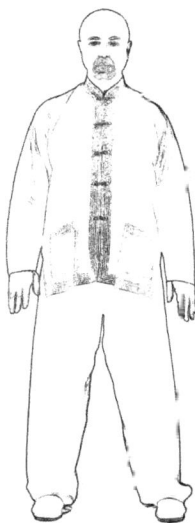

20a side view       20b side view       20c side view

20d side view       20e side view

**20a** The feet and legs remain in the same position. Slowly lower both arms in front of your body with the left hand on top of the right palm, guiding the Qi down to the Lower Dan Tian (area beneath the navel). The thumbs touch gently. Pause in this position for three seconds allowing the Qi to settle.

20b Relax your arms and separate the hands. Slowly scoop your hands up over your head gathering the Qi to the Bai Hui (top of head).

**20c,d,e** Guide Qi down the front of the body to the Lower Dan Tian (area beneath the navel).

## 21. Fluttering over the grass 草上飘

Fluttering or rushing over the grass are movements that represent the Geese walking quickly over the grass. The body is held upright with the eyes looking straight ahead; the legs are straight with the knees locked. Most of the weight is on the heel (similar to race walking) and the ball of the foot is soft and hollow.

*The natural walking movement is light and without force. This way the Qi is smoother and lighter and moves down naturally to the Yong Quan (Kidney K1). Lifting the leg stimulates the Zu San Li (Stomach ST36) which is located 5cm below the knee on the outside of the shin bone. These movements provide all-over Qi circulation and strengthen the Small and Large Orbit.*

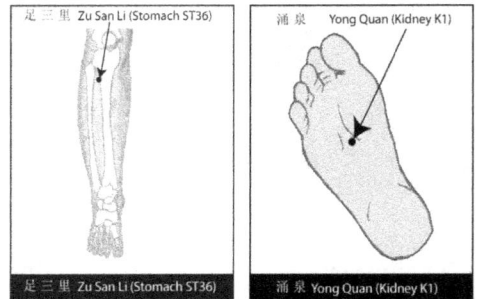

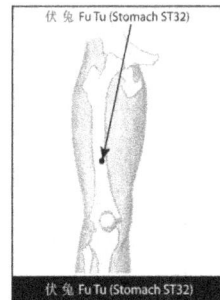

21a      21b

**21a**  Move your bodyweight over the left leg and step forward with the right leg. At the same time the right fingers gently tap (with a loose wrist) the Fu Tu (Stomach ST32) on the middle of the right thigh bone about 12cm above the knee.

**21b**  Then move your bodyweight over the right leg and step forward with the left leg. At the same time the left fingers gently tap the Fu Tu (middle of the thigh bone) of the left leg.

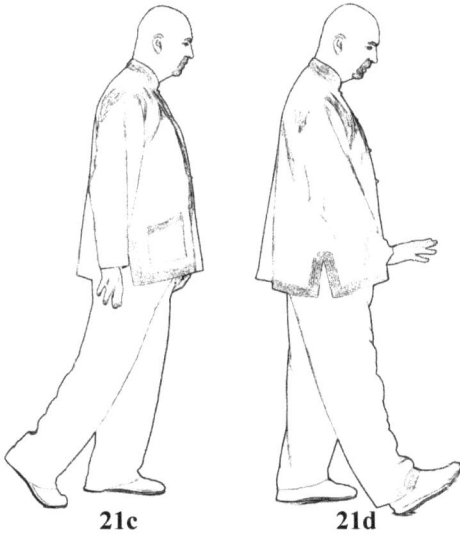

**21c,d** Repeat for a total of nine steps, finishing with your bodyweight on the left leg and right foot forward.

**Benefit:** This sequence of movements benefits the Heart, uterus, ovaries, irregular menstruation and other female health problems.

## 22. Slapping the knees and turning the body 双拍转身

*Slapping the knees moves the Qi from the Lao Gong (middle of palm) to the hands and to the knees to stimulate the Kidney and Stomach Channels.*

**22a** With your bodyweight on the left leg and right foot forward, gently move your bodyweight forward over the right leg and step up with the left foot so both feet are parallel facing the Southern direction. Bend from the waist slightly and gently slap both knees with the palms of both hands.

**22b** Straighten your body and turn 180° to face the Northern direction. Move your bodyweight to the left and pivot on the ball of the right foot turning the heel in as far as feels comfortable.

**22c** With your right toes facing towards the North West direction, move your bodyweight over the right leg and swing the body around in a clockwise direction. Adjust your feet so both are parallel and facing the Northern direction. Eyes are locking straight ahead.

# 23.Crossing the arms 十字臂

23a                              23b

**23a** The feet and legs stay in the same position. Both arms rise up in front of the body, with the right arm closer to the body and both arms crossed at the wrist. This connects the Nei Guan (inner point) in the middle of the outer arm and the Wai Guan (outer point) of the inner arm.

**23b** The right Lao Gong (middle of palm) is gently placed over the left Ku Fang (between the collar bone and the nipple). The left Lao Gong is gently placed over the right Ku Fang. The eyes are looking straight ahead.

# 24. Sending down the Qi 下沉

*Sending down the Qi disperses the negative Qi to the ground through the soles of the feet.*

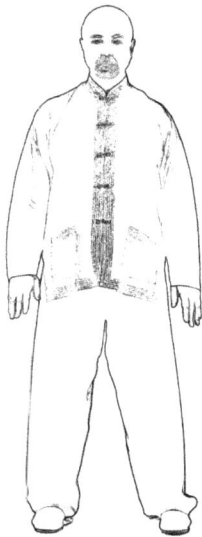

24a          24b          24c          24d          24e

**24a** The feet and legs remain in the same position. Slowly lower both arms in front of the body with the right hand on top of the left palm. Guide the Qi down to the Lower Dan Tian (area beneath the navel). The thumbs touch gently. Pause in this position for three seconds allowing the Qi to settle

**24b** Relax the arms and separate the hands. Slowly scoop up over the head gathering the Qi to the Bai Hui (top of head).

**24c,d,e** Guide the Qi down the front of the body to the Lower Dan Tian (area beneath the navel).

24e side view

## 25.  Fluttering over the grass 草上飄

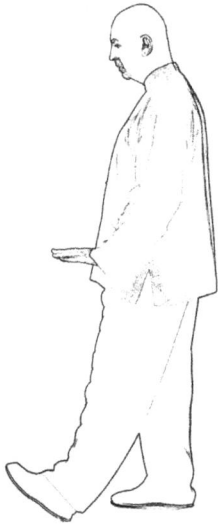

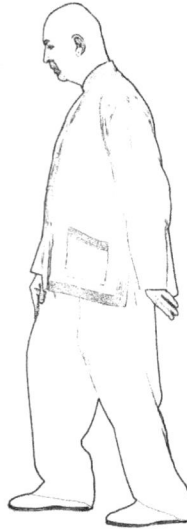

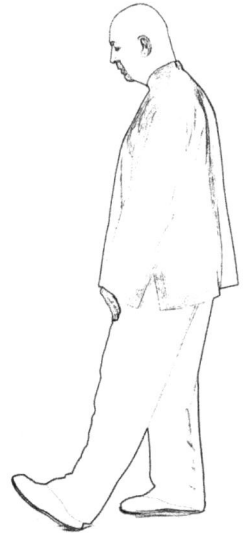

25a                    25b                    25c

**25a**  Move your bodyweight over the right leg and step forward with the left leg. At the same time the left fingers gently tap the left Fu Tu (middle of thigh).

**25b**  Then move your bodyweight over the left leg and step forward with the right leg. At the same time the right fingers gently brush the right Fu Tu (middle of thigh).

**25c**  Repeat for a total of nine steps, finishing with your bodyweight on the right leg and left foot forward.

## 26.  Slapping the knees and turning the body 双拍转身

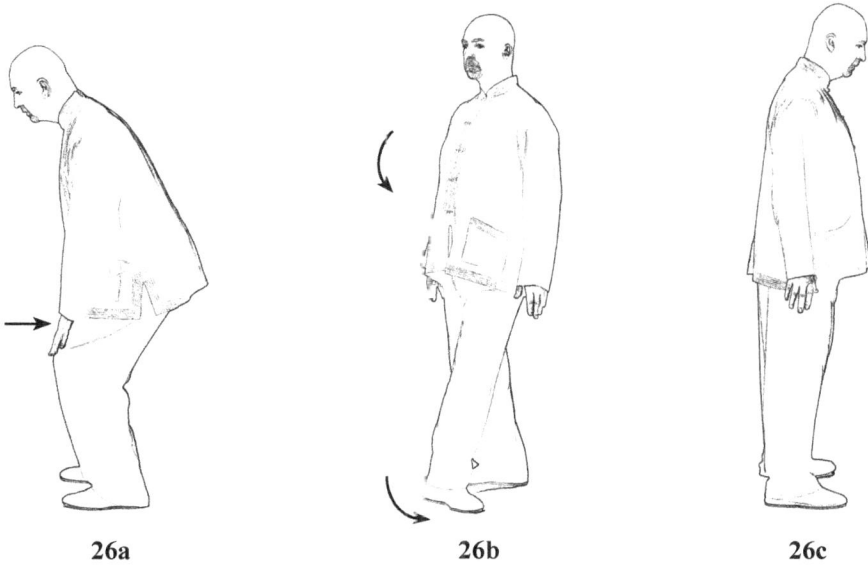

26a                    26b                    26c

**26a**    Your bodyweight is on the right leg and left foot forward, gently move your bodyweight forward over the left leg and step up with the right foot so both feet are parallel and facing the Northern direction. Bend from the waist slightly and gently slap both knees with the palms of both hands.

**26b,c**   Straighten the body and turn 180° to face the Southern direction. Move your bodyweight to the right and pivot on the ball of the left foot turning the heel in as far as feels comfortable. With the right toes facing towards the South West direction, move your bodyweight over the left leg and swing the body around in a counter clockwise direction. Adjust your feet so both are parallel and facing the Southern direction. Eyes are looking straight ahead.

## 27.   Crossing the arms 十字臂

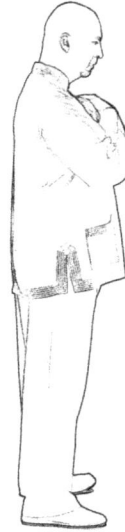

27a                                                      27b

**27a**   The feet and legs stay in the same position with the body facing the Southern direction. Both arms rise up in front of the body, with the left arm closer to the body and both arms crossed at the wrist. This connects the Nei Guan (inner point) in the middle of the outer arm and the Wai Guan (outer point) of the inner arm.


**27b**   The left Lao Gong (middle of palm) is gently placed over the right Ku Fang (between the collar bone and the nipple). The right Lao Gong is gently placed over the left Ku Fang. The eyes are looking straight ahead.

# 28.  Sending down the Qi 下沉

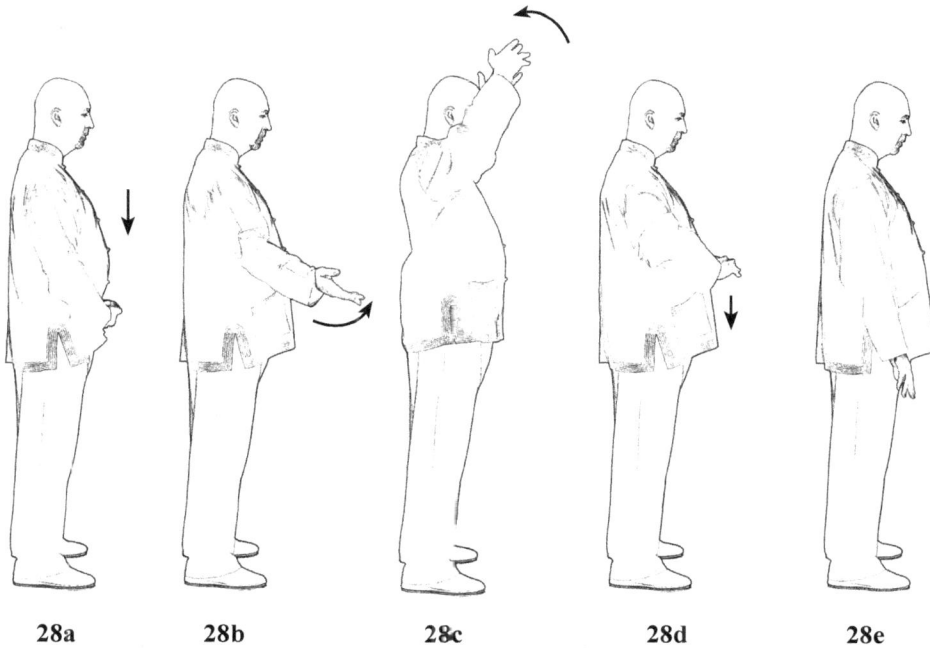

28a        28b        28c        28d        28e

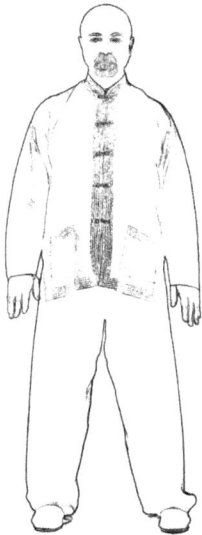

**28a**   The feet and legs remain in the same position. Slowly lower both arms in front of the body with the left palm on top of the right hand. Guide the Qi down to the Lower Dan Tian (area beneath the navel). The thumbs touch gently. Pause in this position for three seconds, allowing the Qi to settle.

**28b,c**  Relax the arms and separate the hands, slowly scoop up over the head gathering the Qi to the Bai Hui (top of head).

**28d,e**  Guide the Qi down the front of the body to the Lower Dan Tian (area beneath the navel).

28e side view

# 29. Slapping the back of the legs 后拍腿

*Slapping behind the knee stimulates and injects Qi into the Three Bladder points.*

**Right slap**

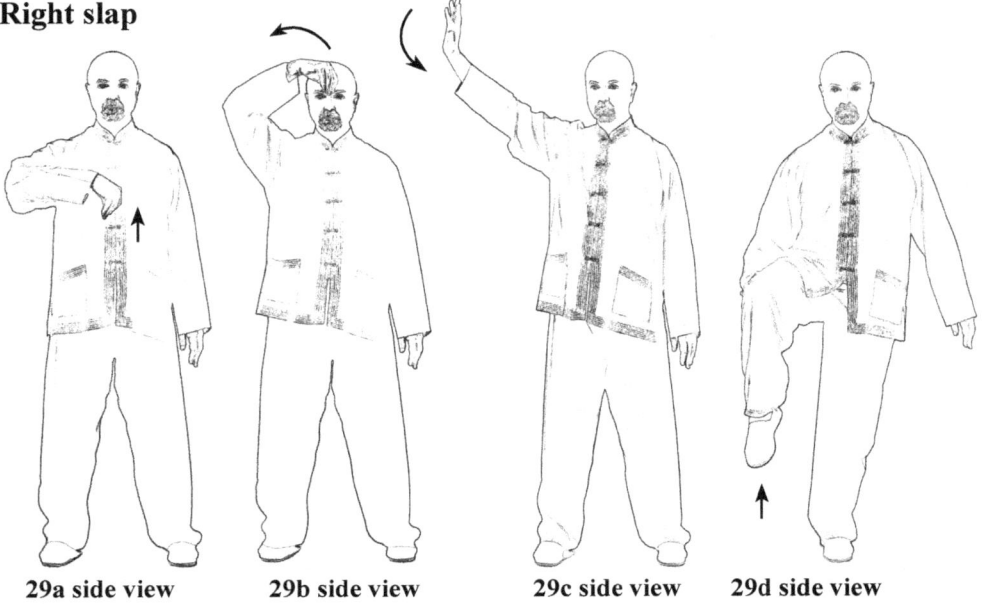

29a side view    29b side view    29c side view    29d side view

29e side view

**29a,b** The feet and legs remain in the same position, facing the Southern direction. The right arm rises up in front of the body, hand relaxed and fingers facing toward the ground. The He Gu (web of hand) scans up the centre line of the body (Conception Vessel) to the Upper Dan Tian (between the eyebrows).

**29c** Keeping the shoulder relaxed, turn palm up and circle arm around to the side and behind the body.

**Benefit:** The slapping and flicking movements strengthen the bones and tendons of the leg and strengthens the autoimmune system.

**Left slap**

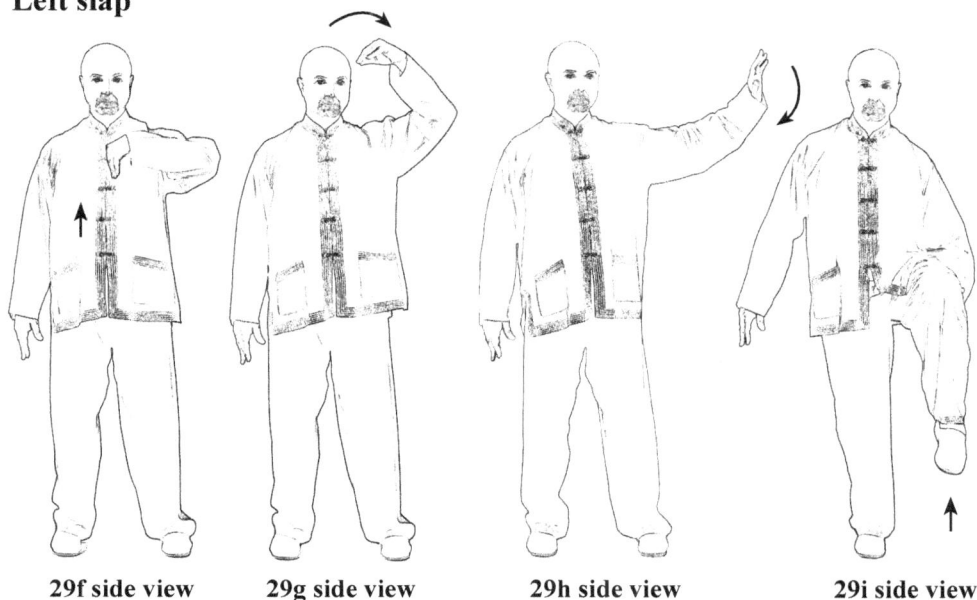

| 29f side view | 29g side view | 29h side view | 29i side view |

**29j side view**

**29f,g** The right arm rises up in front of the body, hand relaxed and fingers facing toward the ground. The He Gu (web of hand) scans up the centre line of the body (Conception Vessel) to the Upper Dan Tian (between the eyebrows).

**29h** Keeping your shoulder relaxed, turn palm up and circle the arm around to the side and behind the body.

**29i** At same time move your bodyweight to the right leg and lift the left knee and with the left hollow palm slap behind the knee, stimulating the Three Bladder points (Fu Xi Bladder BL38, Wei Yang BL39 and Wei Zhong BL40).

**29j,k** The left leg quickly kicks up from the knee. Lower the left leg to the side of the body with feet parallel.

# 30.  Sway three times 跨步三晃

*These swaying movements, with the arms held away from the body, create an energy field around the whole body.*

30a          30b                    30c                           30d

**30a**  The feet and legs remain in the same position, with the body facing the Southern direction. Both arms are positioned away from the body on either side of the buttocks.

**30b,c** Lift the right knee to the height of the waist, pull toes back and straighten the leg, pushing the heel out to the side of the body at an angle of 45°.

**30d**  Place the foot on the ground with the toes facing the Southern direction. Move about 60% of your bodyweight forward over the right leg keeping the knee aligned over the foot; maintain 40% over the left leg. Both feet are firmly grounded to the earth. The arms are still held wide and away from the body.

**Benefit:** This set of movements helps to nourish the reproductive system and benefits the Pancreas and Bladder.

## Left sway

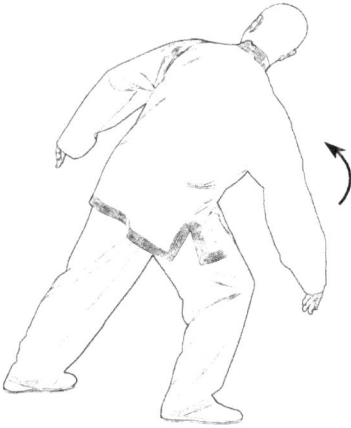

30e

**30e** Move about 80% of your bodyweight forward. Moving from the waist, slightly lean the body forward over the right leg, keeping both feet firmly grounded to the earth. Turn from the waist and sway the body 90° to the left in the counter-clockwise direction. Hips and shoulders are facing the Eastern direction and hands are wide facing either side of the body. The head continues to turn looking to the Northern direction. The left leg is straight, gently stretching the inside of the leg.

## Right sway

**30f,g** Move your bodyweight back onto the left leg and lift the right toes. Pivoting on the right heel, slightly lean back and sway the body 180° to the right in the clockwise direction. Hips and shoulders are facing the Western direction and the hands are facing either side of the body. The head continues to turn looking to the Northern direction. The right leg is straight, gently stretching the inside of the leg.

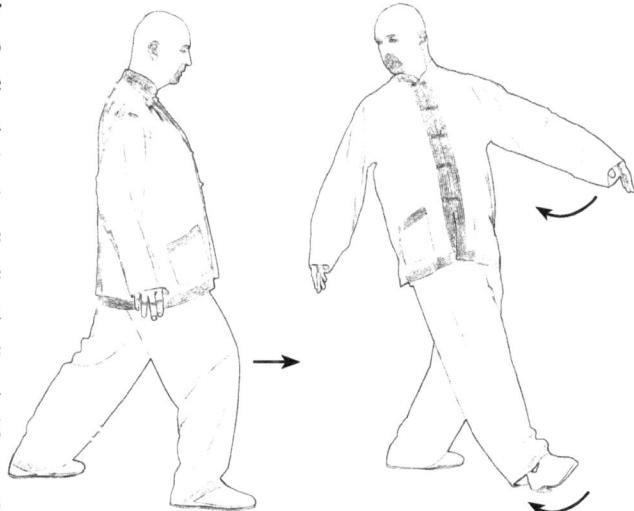

30f          30g

**Continue left and right swaying movements three times (total of six times).**

Move your body back to the central position facing the Southern direction. Your bodyweight is evenly distributed with the right leg forward. The hands remain unchanged on either side of the body.

# 31. Shrinking the body and smoothing the face 缩身修面

*Movements 31-35 nurture and receive Qi which is good for Kidney and brain energy.*

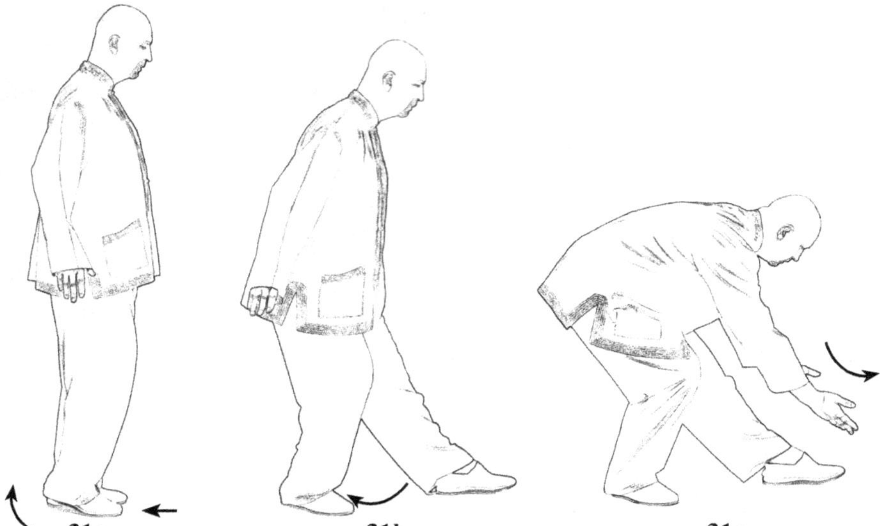

**31a**    **31b**    **31c**

**31a,b** The right leg steps back to the left heel and then further back in a semi-circle. Move your bodyweight back to the right leg. Adjust the left toe and face the body to the Southern direction.

**31c**    Bending forward, scoop your hands up in front of the body, gathering the Qi.

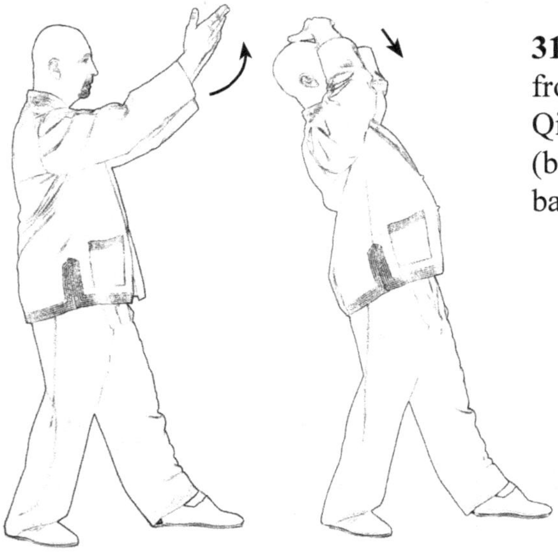

**31d**    **31e**

**31d,e** Lift the hands up in front of the body, lifting the Qi up to the Upper Dan Tian (between the eyebrows). Lean back slightly

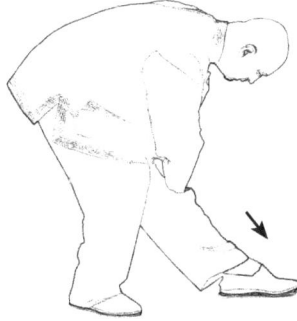

31f                          31g                          31h

**31f** Turn the palms over and with the Lao Gong (middle of palm) guide the Qi down the front of the body.

**31g,h** At waist-height gently bend forward, keeping all your bodyweight sitting over the right leg and guide the Qi down the left leg. The left palm is over the Jie Xi (front of ankle) and the right palm is facing the earth.

**Benefit:** These movements help to regulate blood pressure.

## 32. Scanning the ground 探地

*This movement disperses stale Qi into the earth.*

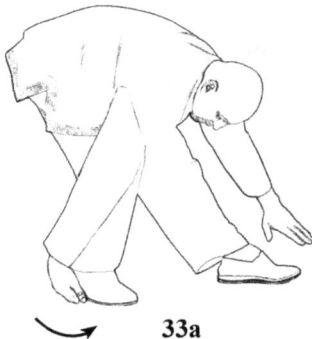

解溪 Jie Xi (Stomach ST41)

解溪 Jie Xi (Stomach ST41)

32a

**32a** Keep your entire bodyweight over the right leg with the left leg extended out in front. The left palm Lao Gong (middle of palm) is over the Jie Xi (front of ankle) and the right palm is facing the earth. Turning from the waist, circle and scan the ground with the right Lao Gong. The eyes follow the hand as it moves behind the right foot to the North West direction.

## 33. Close the palms 合掌

*This movement nurtures the fresh Qi from the earth.*

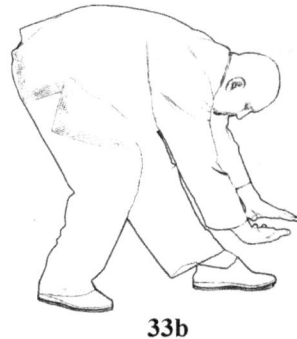

33a                                   33b

**33a** Keep your bodyweight unchanged. The right hand scoops up and gathers the Qi from behind the right foot.

**33b** Turning from the waist and with the palm turned up, move the right hand underneath the left hand, both Lao Gong (middle of palm) are facing each other over the Jie Xi (front of ankle).

## 34. Rubbing the palms 搓掌

*The quick separation of the hands releases and throws out the stale Qi from the head, chest and upper body.*

劳宫 Lao Gong Outer (Pericardium PC8)

劳宫 Lao Gong Outer (Pericardium PC8)

34a                                        34b

**34a** Keep your bodyweight unchanged and sense the Qi between the inner Lao Gong (middle of palm) of both hands.

**34b** Gently push palms closer together, then release the Qi by quickly separating the hands. The Outer Lao Gong (back of hand) of both hands are facing each other.

# 35. Sighting the cloud and watching the fog 寻云看雾

*These movements nurture the Qi from heaven and help stimulate the brain.*

35a                    35b

**35a** Keep your bodyweight unchanged. Turn your body from the waist to face the Southern direction.

**35b** Turn the palms in to face the front and scoop up the Qi while moving your bodyweight forward over the left leg. Straighten the left leg, lifting the right heel and with the right toes touching the ground. The arms rise up lifting the body, holding the Qi in the arms. Shoulders and elbows are relaxed. The eyes are looking up to the sky.

# 36. Stretching back the wings 背翅

*These movements disperse stale Qi from the hands and feet. Qi is received during the movement and is dispersed when the movement is stopped.*

太阳 Tai Yang (extra-ordinary point)

太阳 Tai Yang (extra-ordinary point)

环跳 Huan Tiao (Gallbladder GB30)

环跳 Huan Tiao (Gallbladder GB30)

36a                              36b

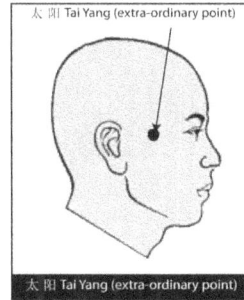

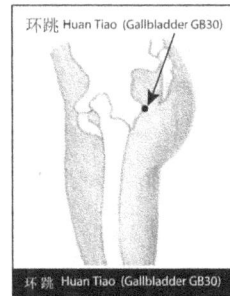

**36a** Your bodyweight remains over the left leg with the leg straight and the right toes just touching the ground. Relax both wrists and form Plum Blossom Claws (four fingers touching together with the thumb) which turn toward the side of the head so the He Gu (web of hand) is connecting to the Tai Yang (an extraordinary point) located at the temple, 3cm back from the eye.

**36b** Lower both arms to the side of the body to hip height with the He Gu (web of hand) facing both Huan Tiao (hip) either side of the buttocks. Pause for two to three seconds.

**Benefit:** This movement helps bladder function.

# 37. Drawing back the arms 回膀

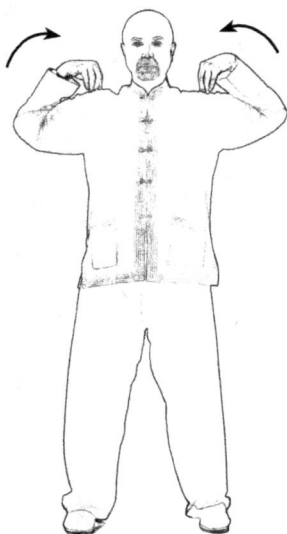

肩 髃 Jian Yu (Large Intestine LI15)

肩 髃 Jian Yu (Large Intestine LI15)

**37a side view**

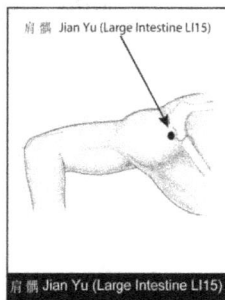

**37a** Your bodyweight remains over the left leg as the right leg steps up placing the right foot parallel with the left foot. Your bodyweight is evenly distributed and the feet are about shoulder-width apart. At the same time relax both Plum Blossom Claws (four fingers touching together with the thumb) and turn both palms up. Gather the Qi with both arms rising up to forehead height, keeping the shoulders and elbows relaxed. Both hands form Plum Blossom Claws (four fingers touching together with the thumb) and fingers touch Jian Yu (Large Intestine LI15) at the tip of the shoulder.

# 38. Injecting the Qi 下贯

*This sequence of movements clears stale Qi from the whole body (five organs – Heart, Spleen, Lungs, Kidney and Liver) into the earth.*

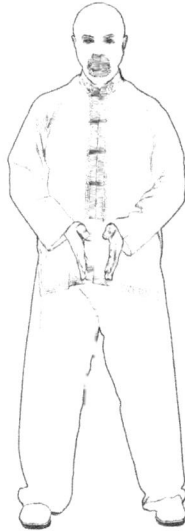

38a side view  38b side view  38c side view

38d side view  38e side view

**38a,b** Keep your bodyweight unchanged, facing and looking to the Southern direction. Relax both Plum Blossom Claws (four fingers touching together with the thumb) and, with the shoulders relaxed, move both arms closer to the centre of the body. The back of the hands face each other and the fingers point to the ground. Lower both arms down the centre of the body to the Lower Dan Tian (area beneath the navel).

**38c,d,e** Separate hands to about the width of the body, circle palms in towards each other gathering the Qi.

**38f side view**   **38g side view**   **38h**   **38i**

**38g,h** Lower the arms to the Lower Dan Tian (area beneath the navel) with palms facing up. Lift arms up higher to Upper Dan Tian (between the eyebrows) and at the same time raise the body lifting the heels off the ground.

**38i** Turn the palms over to face the body and quickly lower arms and body at the same time, bringing your bodyweight firmly on the heels, injecting the Qi down into the face, chest, abdomen and to the Lower Dan Tian (area beneath the navel).

## 39. Rinsing the wings in the water 涮翅

**Rinsing the right wing**

| 39a side view | 39b side view | 39c side view |

**39a,b,c**   Keeping your bodyweight unchanged, place your right palm, with the hand soft and relaxed and the fingers slightly open, facing toward the Liver on the right side of the body. Start to quiver and flutter the hand and gently move it up to the centre of the chest, around to the outside and then up again, circling around the Liver three times.

## Rinsing the left wing

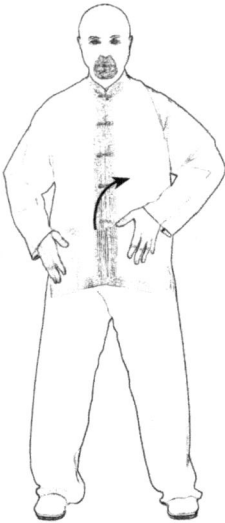 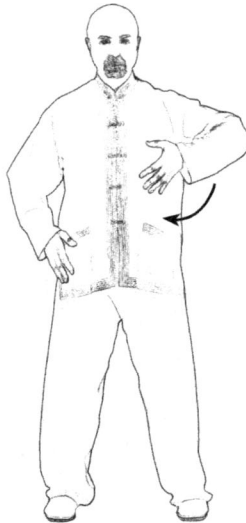 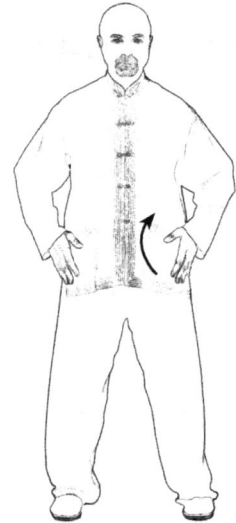

39d side view            39e side view            39f side view

**39d,e,f** With your bodyweight unchanged, the left palm, with the hand soft and relaxed and the fingers slightly open, faces toward the Spleen on the left side of the body. Start to quiver and flutter the hand and gently move it up to the centre of the chest, around to the outside and then up again, circling around the Spleen three times.

**Benefit:** These rinsing movements on both sides of the body help to regulate Heart function and palpitations. Movements 39-41 help nurture the five organs and benefit eyesight.

# 40. Rinsing the arms 涮膀

## Rinsing the right arm

| 40a side view | 40a | 40b | 40c |

**40a** Keep your bodyweight unchanged. The right hand forms the Plum Blossom Claw (four fingers touching together with the thumb). Raise the hand so the fingers touch the right Qi Hu (beneath collar bone). Lift the right elbow to be in line with the shoulder.

**40b,c** Relax the shoulder and elbow and draw the elbow tip back behind the body and then forward. The tip of the elbow is facing the Western direction and drawing a circle in the air. Complete three circles.

## Rinsing the left arm

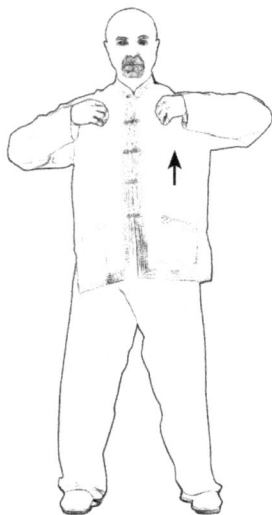 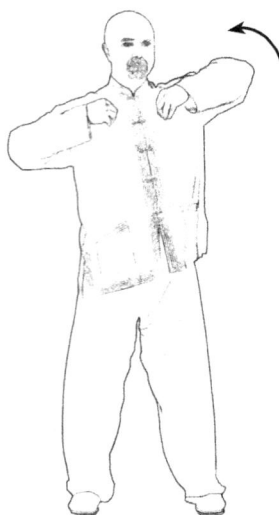 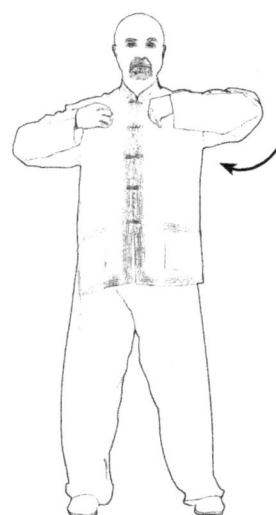

**40e side view**          **40f side view**          **40g side view**

**40e,f**   With the right Plum Blossom Claw (four fingers touching together with the thumb) still touching the right Qi Hu (beneath collar bone), the left hand forms the Plum Blossom Claw and is raised so the fingers touch the left Qi Hu. Lift the left elbow to be in line with the shoulder.

**40g**    Relax shoulder and elbow and draw the elbow tip down and back behind the body and then forward. The tip of the elbow is facing the Eastern direction and drawing a circle in the air. Complete three circles.

**Benefit:** These movements benefit Heart function and gently massage the shoulder and upper back area.

## 41.  Shaking the wings and washing the chest 振翅洗胸

*These movements disperse stale Qi from the five organs (Spleen, Lungs, Kidneys, Liver and Heart) and the gentle rocking motion helps to massage these five organs.*

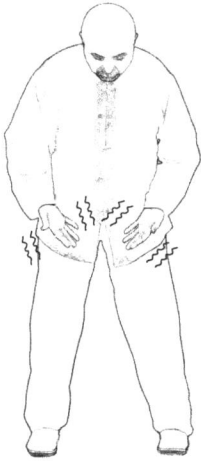
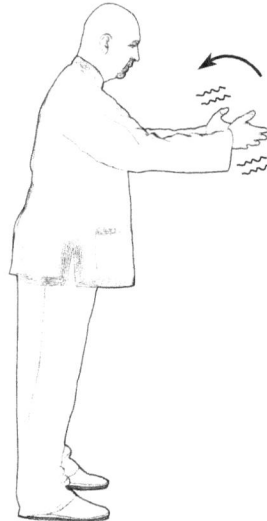
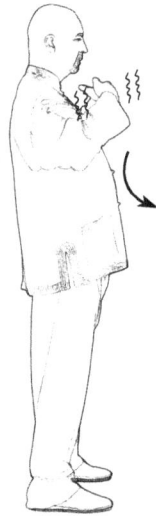

| 41a side view | 41a | 41b | 41c |

**41a,b**  Keep your bodyweight unchanged, facing and looking to the Southern direction. Lower both arms with the palms facing up at the abdomen. Start to quiver and flutter both hands up to chest height as you lean slightly forward with your bodyweight going onto the front of your feet, gently massaging the soles.

**41c**  Move your bodyweight back onto the heels and lean back slightly, gently massaging the soles of the feet. Keep your feet connected to the earth without raising the heels or the toes. Keeping shoulders and elbows relaxed and the palms facing upward, lower your fluttering arms in front of the body to the abdomen.

Continue washing the chest for a total of seven times, rocking backward and forward in a circular movement in coordination with the arms.

**Benefit:** This series of movements aids the digestive system.

## 42. Spreading the wings and washing the head 展翅洗头

*This movement rotates the head in four directions and helps disperse stale Qi.*

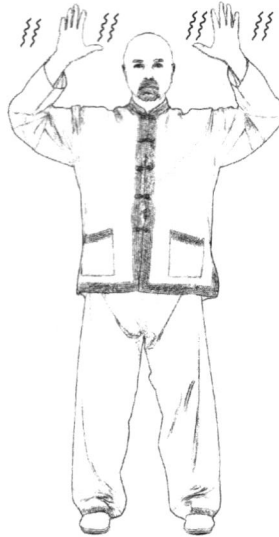 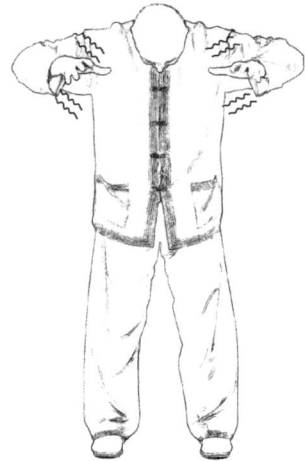

42a                  42b side view         42c side view

**42a**   Keep your bodyweight unchanged. Lower both fluttering arms to the side of the body.

**42b**   Keeping shoulders and elbows relaxed raise both fluttering hands to the side of the head. The thumbs face the temple and are about 5cm away.

**42c**   With the palms facing forward, begin to move the head in a circle. Commence by moving the head down.

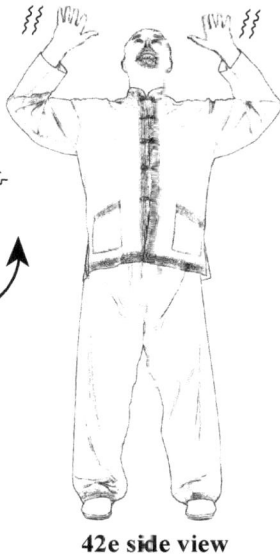

**42d side view**

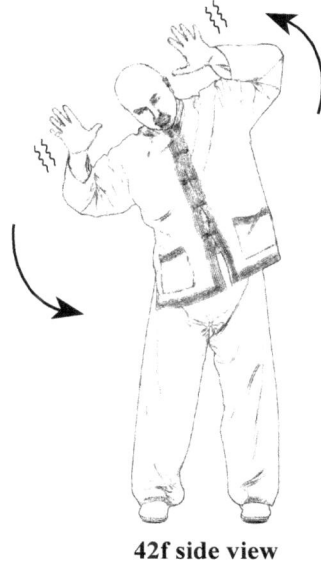

**42e side view**

**42f side view**

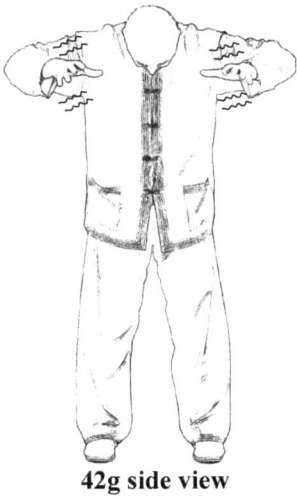

**42g side view**

**42d-g** Relax the left side of the neck and turn the head down to the left, then slightly back facing up to the sky, and around to the right. The fluttering arms follow the circular movement of the head, arms, shoulders and waist. Repeat three times.

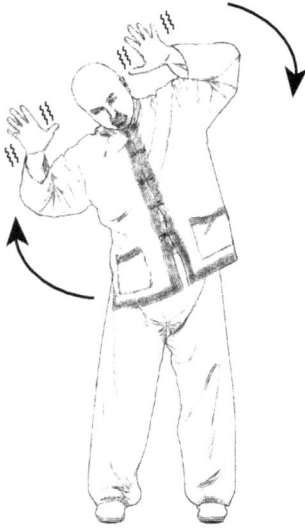

**42h side view**  **42i side view**  **42j side view**

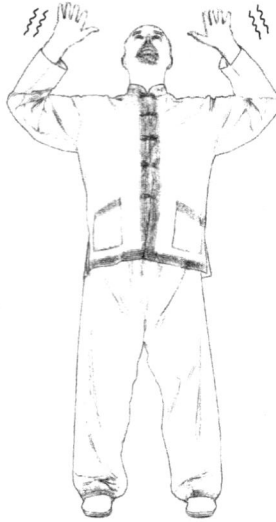

**42k side view**

**42h-k** Then repeat the movement in the opposite direction three times.

**Benefit:** This rotational movement helps stimulate the five senses (Mouth, Nose, Ears, Eyes, Tongue) and benefits the neck, shoulders and throat. This movement is done slowly and comes mainly from the neck with only slight movement from the waist. It is also beneficial for hearing problems and tinnitus

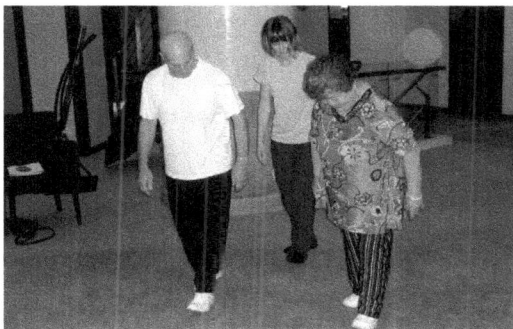
**Fluttering over the grass** 草 上 飄

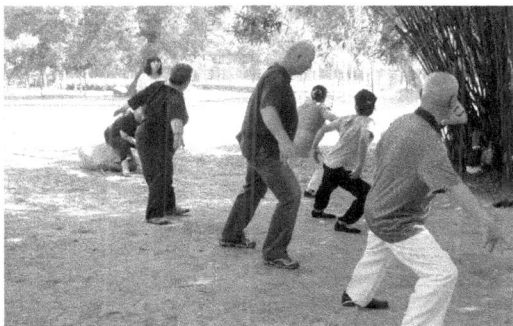
**Sway three times** 跨 步 三 晃

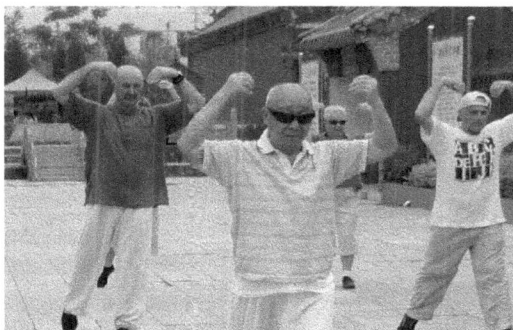
**Stretching back the wings** 背 翅

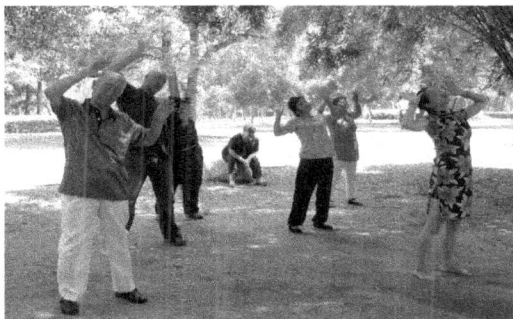
**Spreading the wings and washing the head** 展 翅 洗

## 43. Drawing back the wings 落膀收翅

*In this movement the Yin and Yang Channels are regulated as the hands slowly stop fluttering and move down in front of the body.*

**43a side view**

**43a** Keep your bodyweight unchanged, facing and looking to the Southern direction. Relax the shoulders and elbows and move the arms down in front of the body with the palms facing up and forming the Plum Blossom Claw (four fingers touching together with the thumb) which touches the Da Bao (middle of ribs) at the side of the body. Pause for two to three seconds to allow the Qi to settle.

## 44. Starting to fly 泳动起飞

*In this movement Qi is nurtured as the hands circle up in front of the body and dispersed as the hands circle around the back of the body.*

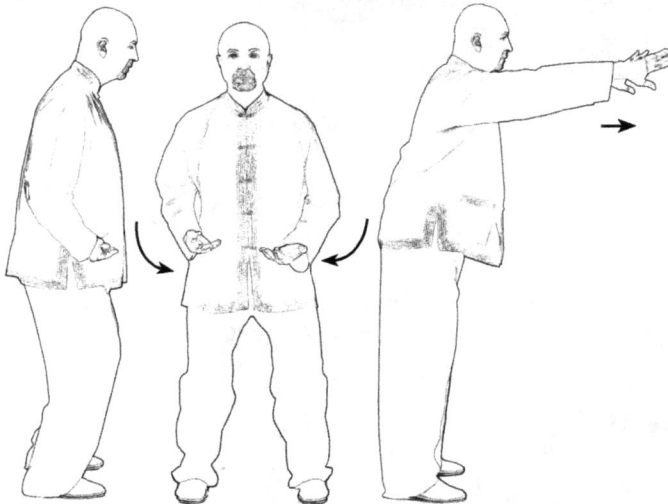

**44a**    **44a side view**    **↑ 44b**

**44a** Keep your bodyweight unchanged. Release the Plum Blossom Claws (four fingers touching together with the thumb) and lower the palms onto the Dai Mai (below the ribs).

**44b** Push the palms out in front to shoulder height and start to flutter the hands gently; at the same time lift your bodyweight up onto the balls of your feet. The hands separate with palms turning outwards at forehead height (Upper Dan Tian) and the fluttering of the hands increases as if starting to fly.

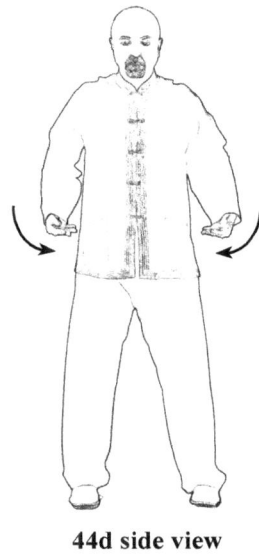

**44b side view**　　　　**44c**　　　　**44d side view**

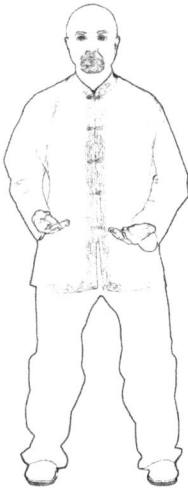

**44e side view**

**44c**　Circle both fluttering arms around to the side of the body.

**44d**　Turn the palms up to rest on the Dai Mai (below the ribs).

**44e**　Your bodyweight is gently dropped onto the heels in coordination with the palms resting below the ribs.

Repeat for a total of seven times

**Benefit:** This movement benefits the digestive system and the chest.

## 45. Pointing to heaven 指天

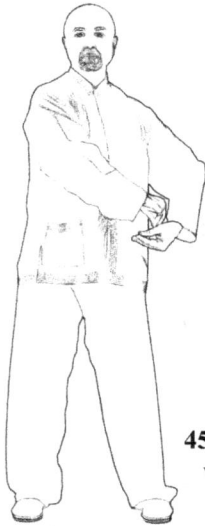

**45a side view**

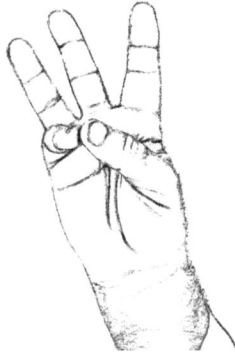

**45b**

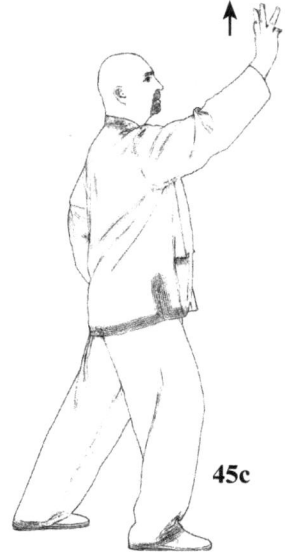

**45c**

**45a** Both hands form Plum Blossom Claws (four fingers touching together with the thumb) and the fingers touch Dai Mai (below the ribs). Keep your bodyweight unchanged. Relax both Plum Blossom Claws and turning from the waist the right hand moves around the front of the body and in a circle underneath the left hand.

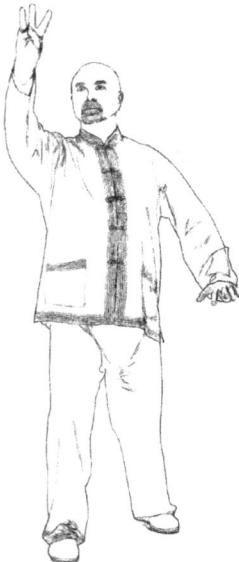

**45c side view**

**45b** At the same time, the right fingers form together with the tip of the thumb Shao Shang (Lung LU11) touching the tip of the small finger Shao Chong (Heart HT9).

**45c** Move your bodyweight over the left leg and step forward with the right leg. Maintain about 60% of your bodyweight over the right leg and 40% over the left leg, keeping both feet firmly grounded. Your right arm moves in coordination with body movement forward and swings up to over the head, keeping shoulders and elbow relaxed. The thumb and small finger are touching and the other three fingers are pointing to heaven. Stay in this position for three seconds looking at the right hand. At the same time, the left hand pushes down to the left with the fingers pointing forward at waist height.

**Benefit**: In this movement the fingers are pointing like an antenna connecting to the heaven. It improves brain function, intelligence and nervous system function.

# 46. Drawing circles on the earth 划地

*In this movement we are nurturing the Qi we gathered from the 'antenna' in the 'pointing to heaven' movement and the Kunlun belt (the area around the outside of the foot between the depression above the heel and the front of the foot) is receiving the Qi from the hand. The opposite hand faces the earth and is dispersing the Qi.*

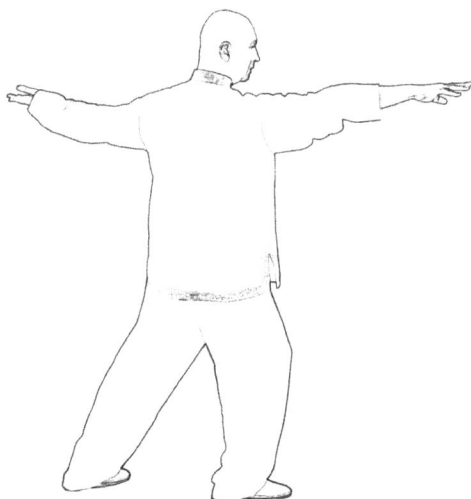

46a

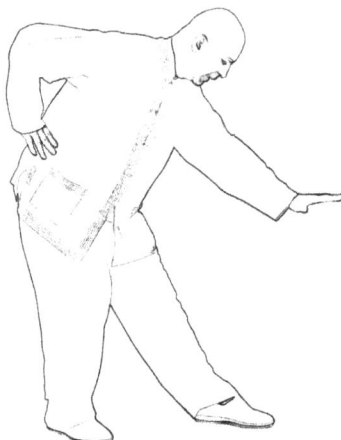

46b

**46a**    Maintain about 60% of your bodyweight over the right leg and 40% over the left leg, and keep both feet firmly grounded. Relax right fingers and lower the arm to shoulder height with the palm facing the ground and the fingers pointing towards the Southern direction. At the same time, raise the left arm to shoulder height with the palm facing to the sky and fingers pointing to the Northern direction. Move your bodyweight back onto the left leg and step backwards with the right leg. At the same time, rotate both arms in coordination, similar to turning a large wheel.

**46b**    Move your bodyweight back onto the right leg and pushing the bottom back, bend forward from the waist. The right hand pushes down and up sitting at waist height. The left arm pushes down with the palm over the left foot. The eyes are looking at the hand.

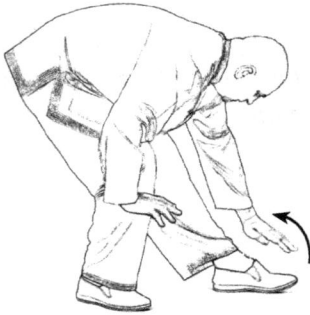

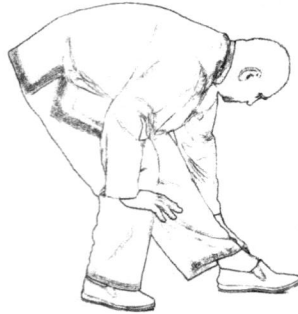

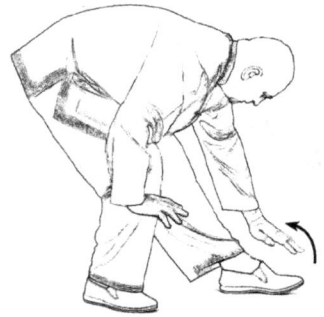

| 46c | 46d | 46e |

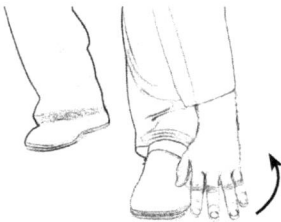

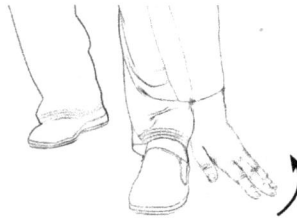

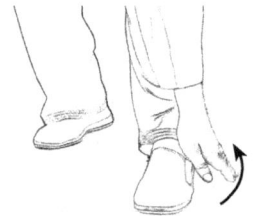

| 46c side closeup | 46d side closeup | 46e side closeup |

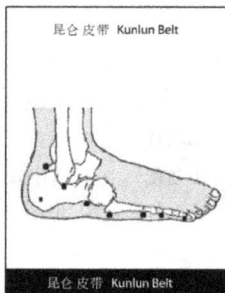

昆仑 皮带  Kunlun Belt

昆仑 皮带  Kunlun Belt

**46c,d,e** Moving from the waist and arm, the left palm draws a circle in a counter-clockwise direction around the outside of the left foot and back again three times. At the same time the right hand is facing towards the earth.

## 47. Turning the body and drawing circles on the earth 转身划地

*The right hand is nurturing the Qi into the Kunlun belt while the left hand is dispersing Qi.*

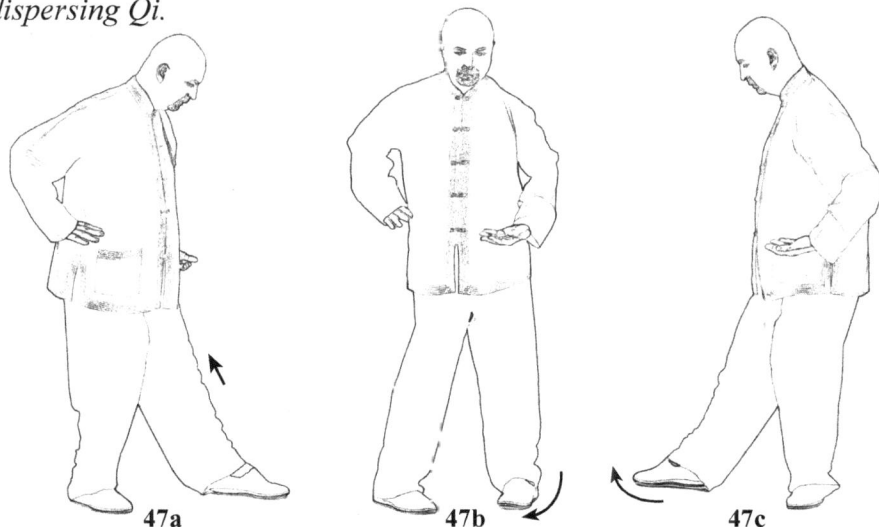

47a      47b      47c

**47a**      Turn the left palm up to face the sky and gently lift the upper body from the waist as the left palm draws up the outside of the leg to rest on the waist with the fingers pointing forward. The right palm is facing upwards. The body is standing upright facing the Southern direction.

**47b**      Turn the body 180° to face the Northern direction. Move your bodyweight back onto the right leg and pivoting on the left heel hook the left toe in as far as feels comfortable.

**47c**      Move your bodyweight back onto the left leg and pivot on the right heel turning the right toe out

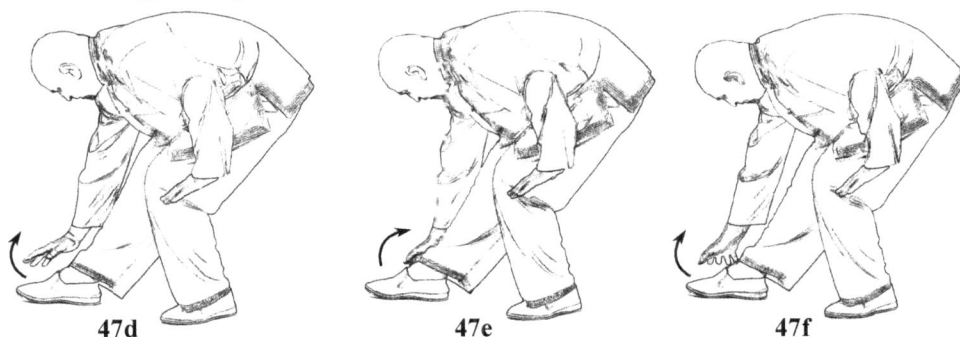

47d      47e      47f

**47d,e,f** Pushing the bottom back and bending forward from the waist, lower the right arm with the palm over the right foot. The eyes are looking at the hand. Moving from the waist and arm, the right palm draws a circle in a clockwise direction around the outside of the right foot and back again three times. At the same time the left palm is facing towards the earth

# 48.   Holding up the Qi 捧气

*In this movement we are gathering external Qi with both hands to create a large Qi ball. According to Master Chen, the posture is similar to that of a turtle. The holding and balancing of the Qi ball harmonises and regulates the Qi of the whole body*

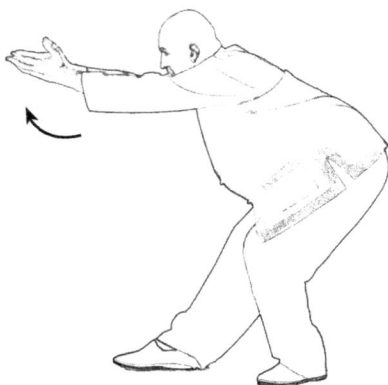

**48a**

**48a**     Keeping your bodyweight over the left leg and bent over from the waist, lift both arms up in front of your body with both palms facing the sky. Gently push your bottom back slightly, keeping the shoulders and elbows relaxed. Look at your hands which are in front of the Upper Dan Tian (area between the eyebrows).

# 49.   Sending back the Qi 归回

*In this movement we are refining and balancing the Qi of the whole body. The Qi moves through the three Dan Tians from left to right and front to back.*

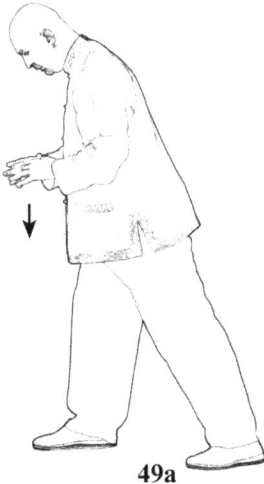

49a

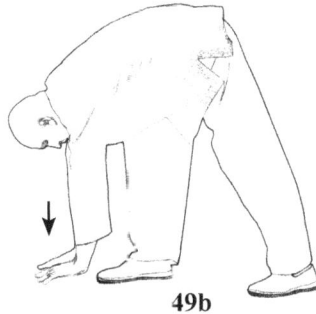

49b

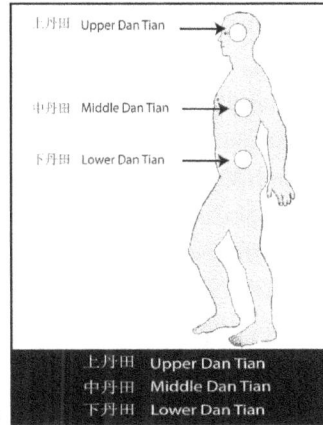

| 上丹田 Upper Dan Tian |
| 中丹田 Middle Dan Tian |
| 下丹田 Lower Dan Tian |

| 上丹田 Upper Dan Tian |
| 中丹田 Middle Dan Tian |
| 下丹田 Lower Dan Tian |

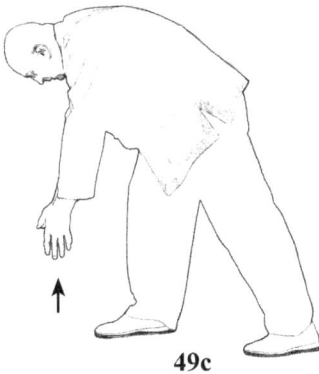

49c

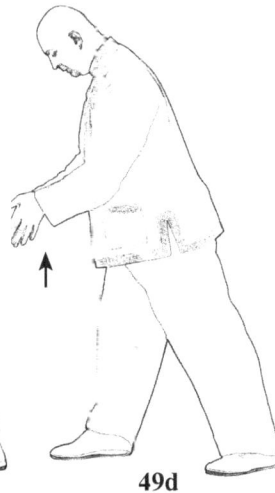

49d

**49a,b** Keeping your bodyweight over the left leg and bent over from the waist, move your bodyweight forward over the right leg and gently lift your upper body from the waist. Keep the left foot firmly grounded to the earth. For people with poor flexibility, simply lift the back heel off the ground. Turn both hands over with the palms facing the earth and then gently push the bottom back and bend forward from the waist. Looking between your hands, the fingers face each other and are soft and relaxed. Gently extend the arms and press down in front of the right foot sending back the Qi.

**49c,d** Gently lift the upper body from the waist while looking at the hands, keeping the fingers separated and relaxed and pointing to the ground. The fingers are slightly tense drawing up the energy from the earth.

Repeat down and up movements for a total of three times.

**Benefit:** This movement improves Gall Bladder function.

# 50. Circular Steps 连环步

Gently lift the upper body from the waist, facing the Northern direction.

The circular steps are three sets of three stepping movements, coordinating arms and legs and gently swaying the body from side-to-side. The movement is similar to the classic drunken swordsmen from the Chinese Martial Arts. The stepping movements are clear, precise and solidly grounded to the earth; with each step forward the heel is placed down quickly creating a little stumbling movement.

*This series of three stepping movements nurture Qi through the Lao Gong (middle of palm) with the circular stepping and disperses Qi with the quick separation of the hands. The movements also stimulate the Qi in and out of the Yong Quan (soles of the foot) and strengthen the Qi of the Large Orbit.*

**1st three steps**

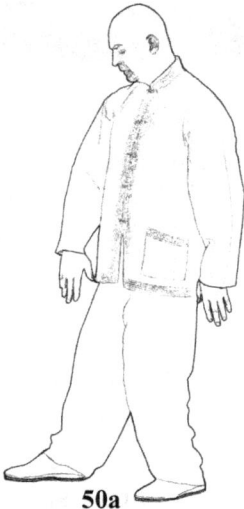 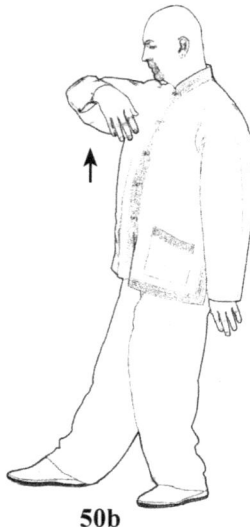 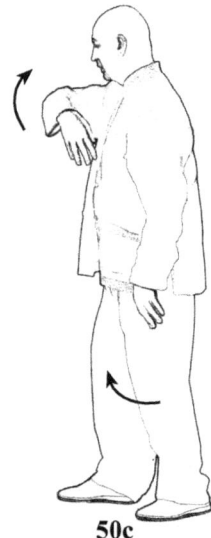

50a                 50b                 50c

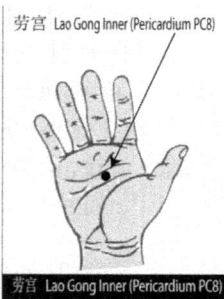

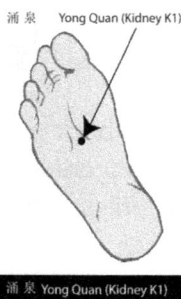

**50a** Shifting your bodyweight over the right leg, bend the right elbow and lift the right hand up the centre line (Ren Channel) of the body. The hand is soft and relaxed with the fingers pointing to the ground.

**50b,c** The He Gu (web of hand) is drawing up the Ren Channel to the Upper Dan Tian (between the eyebrows). At the same time, turn the body from the waist 45° to the right facing the North East direction and lift the left leg in preparation for stepping across in front of the right foot.

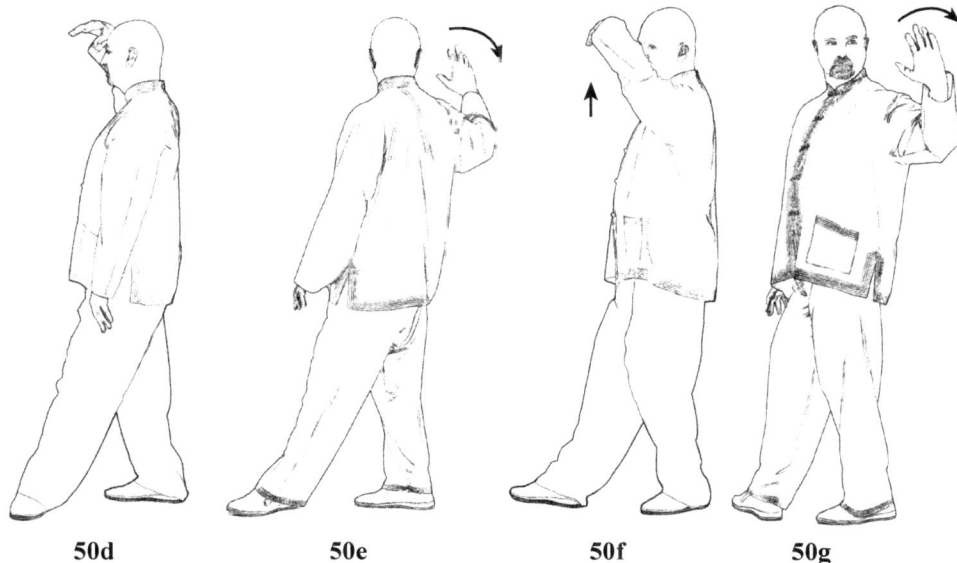

**50d** **50e** **50f** **50g**

**50d,e**  Place the left heel on the ground with the left toes facing 45° to the North West direction. The eyes follow the right hand as it circles around to the side of the body as your bodyweight is moved forward over the left leg.

**50f**  The left hand moves in front of the Lower Dan Tian (area beneath the navel). Bend the left elbow and lift the left hand. The He Gu (web of hand) is drawing up the Ren Channel to the Upper Dan Tian (between the eyebrows). At the same time turn the body from the waist 45° to the left to face the North West direction and lift the right leg stepping across in front of the left foot. Place the right heel on the ground with the right toes facing 45° to the North East direction.

**50g**  The eyes follow the left hand as it circles around to the side of the body as your bodyweight is moved forward over the right leg.

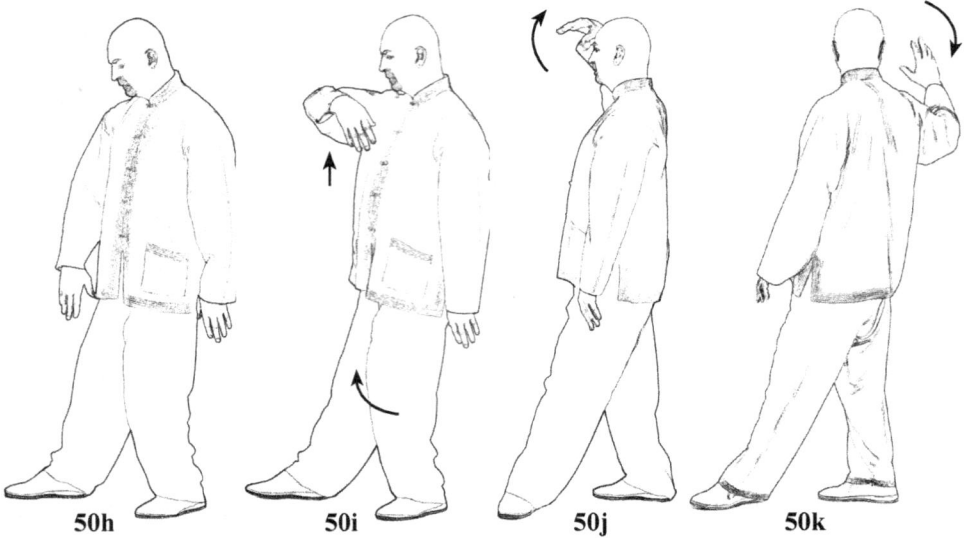

**50h**      **50i**      **50j**      **50k**

**50h,i**  The right hand moves in front of the Lower Dan Tian (area beneath the navel). Bend the right elbow and lift the right hand. The He Gu (web of hand) is drawing up the Ren Channel to the Upper Dan Tian (between the eyebrows). At the same time, turn the body from the waist 45° to the right to face the North East direction and lift the left leg stepping across in front of the right foot. Place the left heel on the ground with the left toes facing 45° to the North West direction.

**50j,k**  The eyes follow the left hand as it circles around to the side of the body as your bodyweight is moved forward over the right leg.

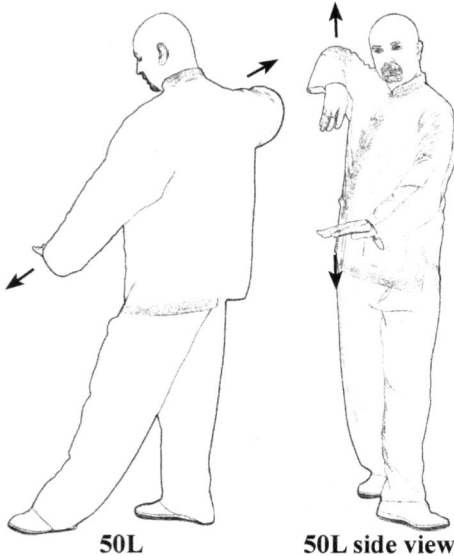

**50L**      **50L side view**

**50L**  After the third step, maintain your bodyweight on the right leg. Rotate the hands one full rotation towards the body, the left hand closer and the right hand on the outside. Quickly separate both hands, the left palm pushes out in front of the Dan Tian towards the ground. At the same time, bend the right elbow and push it back and up. The right fingers are pointing toward the left He Gu (web of hand) and the eyes are looking at the left hand in front of the Lower Dan Tian (area beneath the navel).

## 2nd three steps

**50m**  The left hand moves in front of the Dan Tian at the abdomen. Bend the left elbow and lift the left hand. The He Gu (web of hand) is drawing up the Ren Channel to the Upper Dan Tian (between the eyebrows). At the same time, turn the body from the waist 45° to the left to face the North West direction and lift the right leg stepping across in front of the left foot. Place the right heel on the ground with the right toes facing 45° to the North East direction.

50m    50n

**50n**  The eyes follow the left hand as it circles around to the side of the body as your bodyweight is moved forward over the right leg.

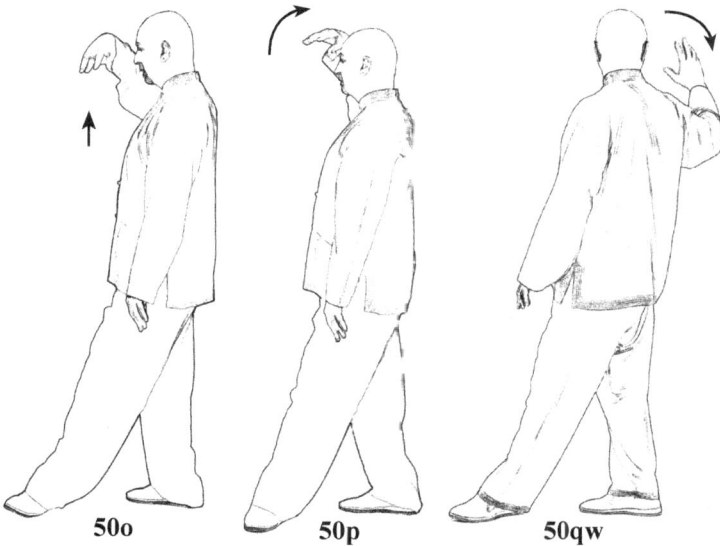

**50o,p**  The right hand moves in front of the Lower Dan Tian (area beneath the navel). Bend the right elbow and lift the right hand. The He Gu (web of hand) is drawing up the Ren Channel to the Upper Dan Tian (between the eyebrows). At the

50o    50p    50qw

same time, turn the body from the waist 45° to the right to face the North East direction and lift the left leg stepping across in front of the right foot. Place the left heel on the ground with the left toes facing 45° to the North West direction.

**50q**  The eyes follow the right hand as it circles around to the side of the body at the waist as your bodyweight is moved forward over the left leg.

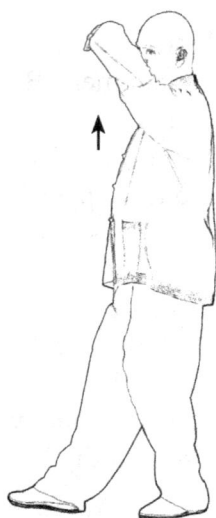 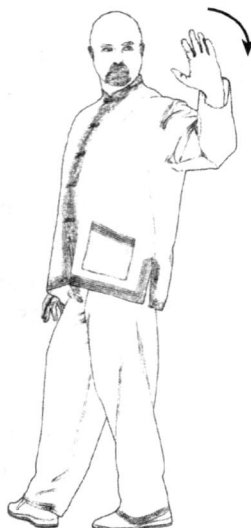 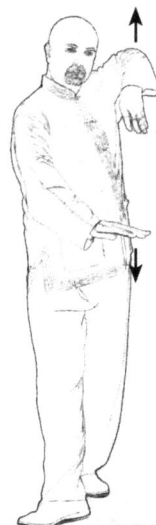

**50r**               **50s**               **50 t side view**

**50r** The left hand moves in front of the Lower Dan Tian (area beneath the navel). Bend the left elbow and lift the left hand. The He Gu (web of hand) is drawing up the Ren Channel to the Upper Dan Tian (between the eyebrows). At the same time turn the body from the waist 45° to the left to face the North West direction and lift the right leg stepping across in front of the left foot.

**50s** Place the right heel on the ground with the right toes facing 45° to the North East direction.

**50t** After the third step maintain your bodyweight on the left leg. Rotate the hands towards the body, with the right hand closer to the body and the left hand on the outside. Quickly separate both hands. The right palm pushes out in front of the Lower Dan Tian (area beneath the navel) towards the ground. At the same time, bend the left elbow and push with the elbow pointing back and up. The left fingers are pointing towards the right He Gu (web of hand) and the eyes are looking at the right hand in front of the Lower Dan Tian (area beneath the navel).

## 3rd three steps

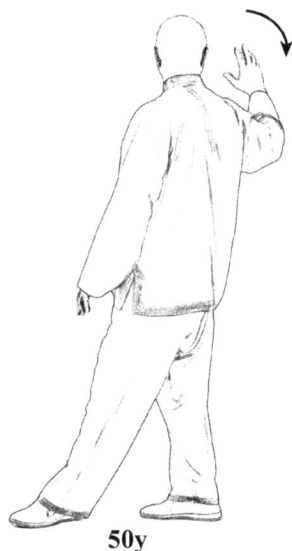

50u      50v      50w      50x

50y

**50u**  Shifting your bodyweight over the right leg, bend the right elbow and lift the right hand up the centre line (Ren Channel) of the body. The hand is soft and relaxed with the fingers pointing to the ground.

**50v,w**  The He Gu (web of hand) is drawing up the Ren Channel to the Upper Dan Tian (between the eyebrows). At the same time, turn the body from the waist 45° to the right facing the North East direction and lift the left leg in preparation for stepping across in front of the right foot.

**50x,y**  Place the left heel on the ground with the left toes facing 45° to the North West direction. The eyes follow the right hand as it circles around to the side of the body as your bodyweight is moved forward over the left leg.

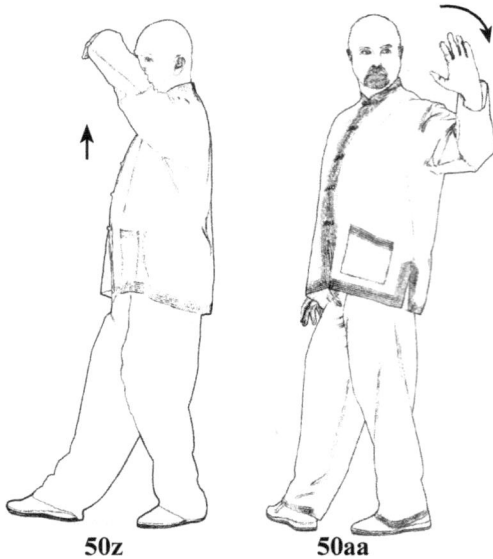

**50z** The left hand moves in front of the Lower Dan Tian (area beneath the navel). Bend the left elbow and lift the left hand. The He Gu (web of hand) is drawing up the Ren Channel to the Upper Dan Tian (between the eyebrows). At the same time turn the body from the waist 45° to the left to face the North West direction and lift the right leg stepping across in front of the left foot. Place the right heel on the ground with the right toes facing 45° to the North East direction.

**50aa** The eyes follow the left hand as it circles around to the side of the body as your bodyweight is moved forward over the right leg.

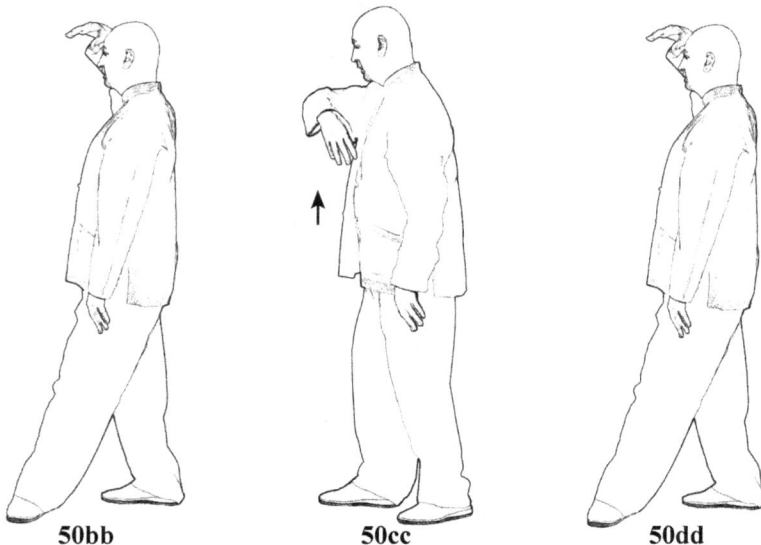

**50bb-dd** The right hand moves in front of the Lower Dan Tian (area beneath the navel). Bend the right elbow and lift the right hand. The He Gu (web of hand) is drawing up the Ren Channel to the Upper Dan Tian (between the eyebrows). At the same time, turn the body from the waist 45° to the right to face the North East direction and lift the left leg stepping across in front of the right foot.

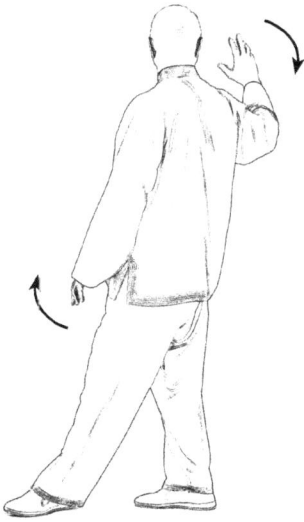
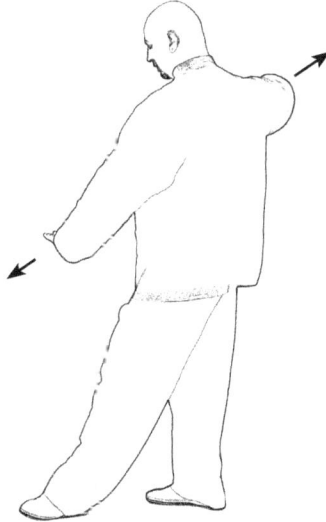
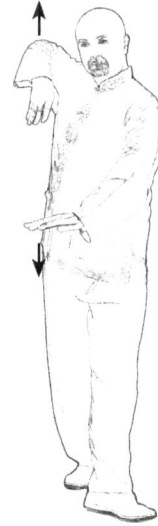

**50ee**                     **50ff**                          **50ff side view**

**50ee** Place the left heel on the ground with the left toes facing 45° to the North West direction.

**50ff** After the third step maintain your bodyweight on the right leg. Rotate the hands towards the body with the left hand closer to the body and the right hand on the outside. Quickly separate both hands, and push the left palm out in front of the Lower Dan Tian (area beneath the navel) towards the ground. At the same time, bend the right elbow and push with the elbow pointing back and up. The right fingers are pointing towards the left He Gu (web of hand) and the eyes are looking at the left hand in front of the Lower Dan Tian (area beneath the navel).

# 51. The hawk turns around 鹞子翻身

*In this movement Qi rises up to the head when the hands circle above which improves brain function and intelligence. The Qi descends when the hands circle down in the squatting position.*

**51a**                       **51b**                      **51c**

**51a,b** Moveyour bodyweight forward over the left leg and lift the right heel. Keep the shoulders and elbows relaxed and lift both arms up in a circle over the head.

**51c**   Pivoting on the right toe hook the right heel in as far as feels comfortable with the foot facing in the South West direction. Gently move your bodyweight over the right leg and at the same time pivot on the left toe turning the whole body 180° to face the Southern direction. The arms continue to swing down in front of the body to the waist.

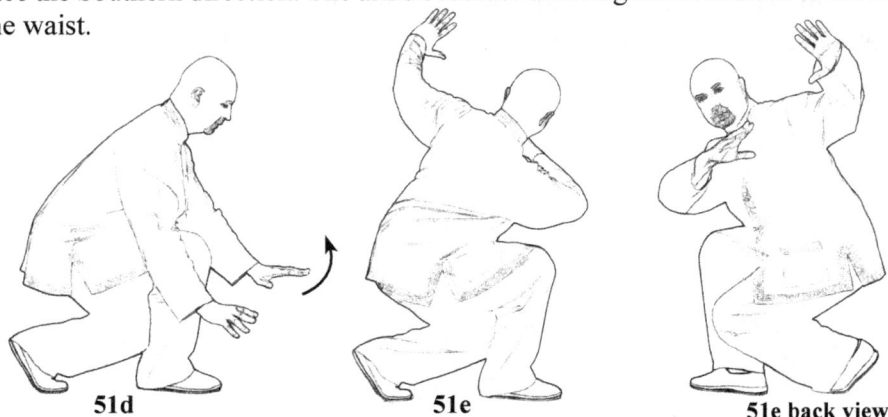

**51d**                      **51e**                   **51e back view**

**51d**   Bend both knees and squat down as far as feels comfortable lowering your bodyweight over the right leg.

**51e** Both arms swing up to the left facing the North Eastern direction to the height of the forehead. The right fingers are pointing towards the left He Gu (web of hand). Eyes are looking at the left hand.

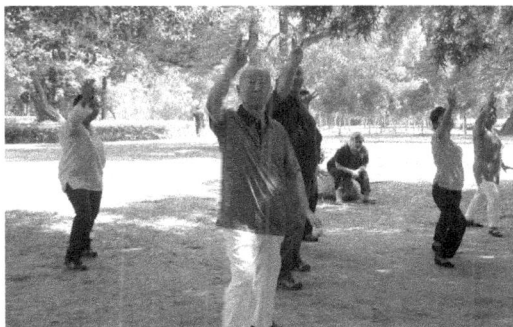
Pointing to heaven 指 天

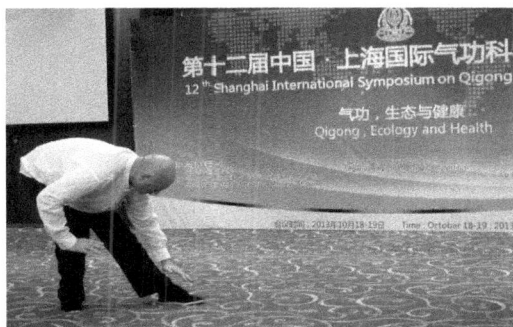
Drawing circles on the earth 划 地

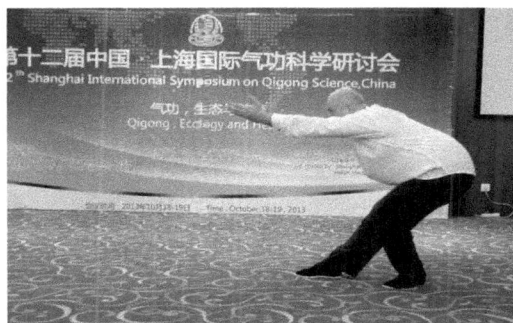
Holding up the Qi 捧 气

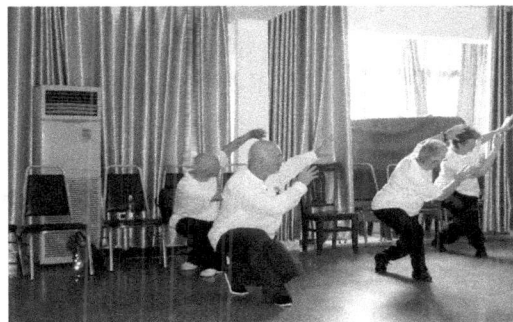
The hawk turns around 鹞 子 翻 身

## 52. Vibrating the shoulders 弹膀

*Movements 52 and 53 release toxins from the chest. The vibrating movements with the palms facing the ground receive Yin Qi from the earth.*

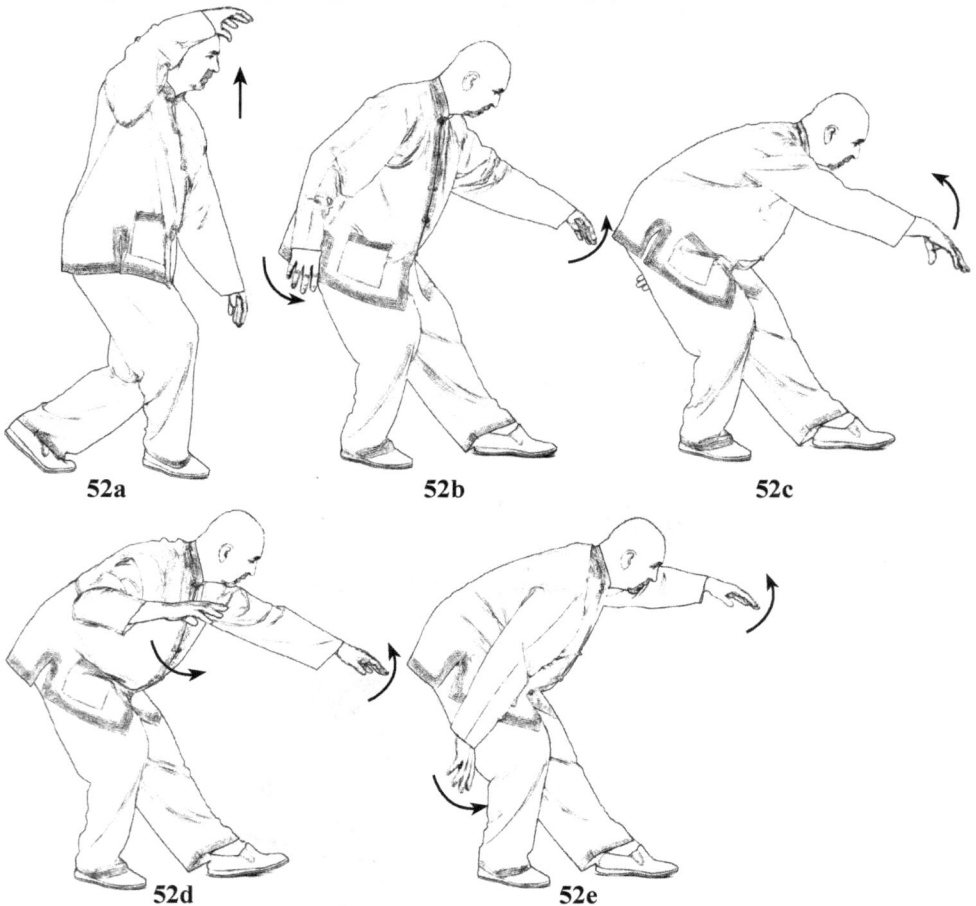

**52a** Gently move your bodyweight forward over the right leg and straighten the right knee to lift the body slightly. The right hand moves up in front of the body connecting the He Gu (web of hand) with the Upper Dan Tian (between eye brows). At the same time the left leg starts to move forward.

**52b-e** The left leg steps forward with the toes just touching the ground and the body is bent forward at an angle of 45°. Lower your arms in front of the body and start to flutter and quiver the arms and hands. Moving from the shoulders and keeping the elbows relaxed, lift the right fluttering arm up and around in a circle and at the same time, alternate the left fluttering arm up and around in a circle. This counts as one rotation. Vibrate the arms for a total of seven rotations.

**Benefit:** These movements are beneficial to the Pancreas and can improve diabetes.

# 53. Penetrating the fog 遮霧

*These movements receive Yang Qi from the sky.*

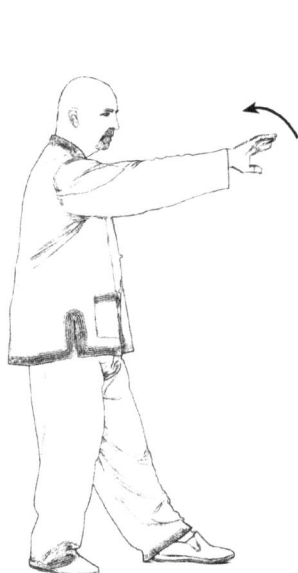

53a

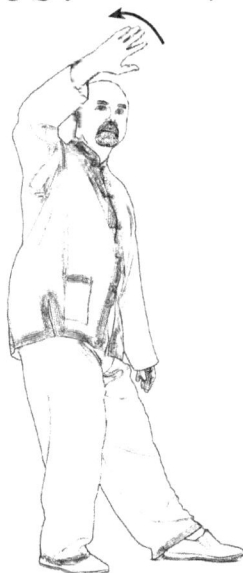

53b

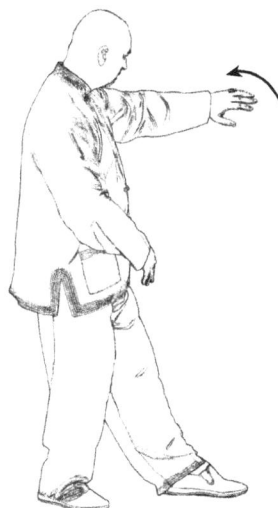

53c

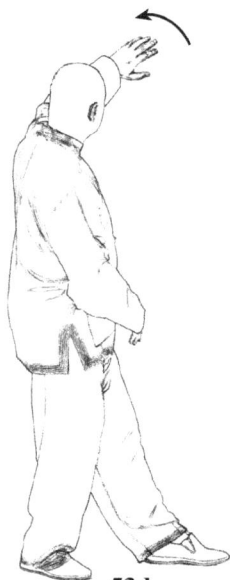

53d

**53a,b** Keep your bodyweight unchanged with the weight on your right leg and the left toe just touching the ground. After completing the seventh rotation with the left hand, slowly lift the upper body from the waist as the right fluttering arm rises in a big arc with the palm turned out to gather the Heaven Qi from the sky. The eyes follow the hand.

**53c,d** Lift the upper body slightly higher as the left fluttering arm rises in a big arc with the palm turned out to gather the Heaven Qi from the sky. The eyes follow the hand. Both hands circle around in front of the body with the palms facing the Lower Dan Tian (area beneath the navel).

# 54. Facing the wind and flying up 看风上飞

*In these movements we are receiving and nurturing Qi through the Lao Gong (middle of palm) when the hands and bodyweight are drawn back, and dispersing Qi as the arms and bodyweight are moved forward. An essential part of this movement is to close the arm pits as the arms pull in and to open the arm pits when the arms push out*

**Face the wind to the left**

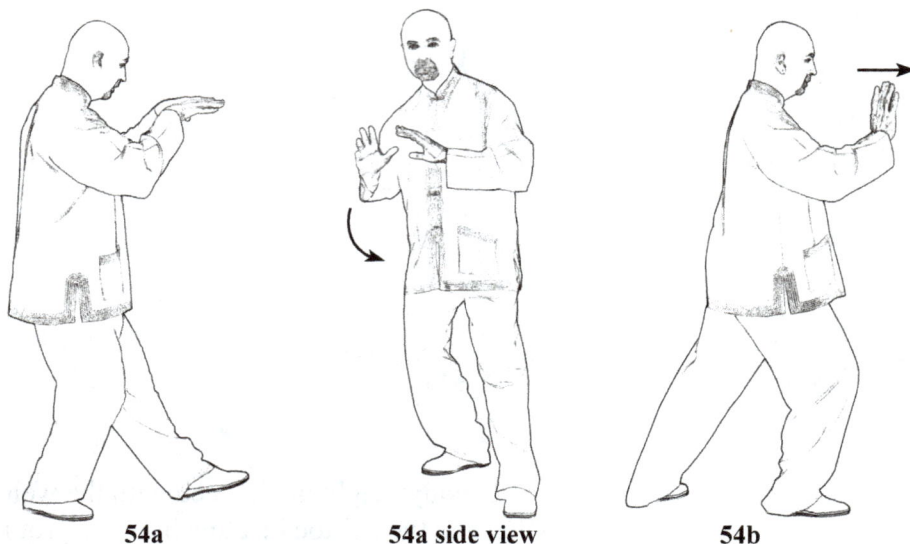

| 54a | 54a side view | 54b |

**54a**  Keeping your shoulders and elbows relaxed, lift both arms in front of the body; the wrists are relaxed and the fingers are pointing to the ground. Bend the elbows and draw both hands back with the He Gu (web of hands) facing towards the Qi Hu (beneath collar bone). With your bodyweight on the right leg, pivot on the ball of the left foot turning the heel in and moving the body slightly to face the South East direction.

**54b**  Move your bodyweight over the left leg and step forward with the right leg facing the Southern direction and move forward with about 60% of your weight over the right leg and 40% over the left leg. At the same time, circle both arms down slightly to the left and push arms up and around to face the wind in coordination with the movement forward. Extend your arms keeping elbows relaxed and arms rounded with hands slightly higher than the shoulders. The He Gu (web of hand) of both hands are facing each other and the hands are soft and relaxed.

# Face the wind to the right

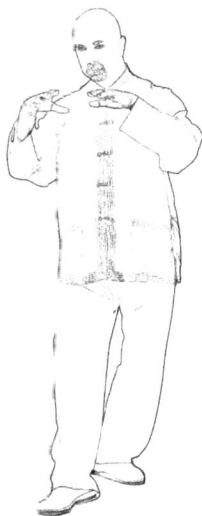

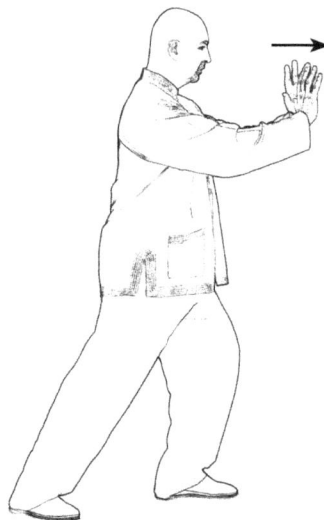

54c            54c side view           54d

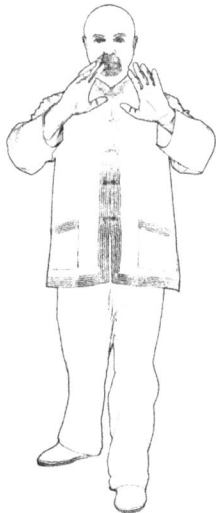

**54c** Keeping shoulders and elbows relaxed lift both arms in front of body, the wrist are relaxed and the fingers pointing to the ground. Bend the elbows and draw both hands back with the He Gu (web of hand) facing forwards the Qi Hu (beneath collar bone). With your bodyweight on the left leg, pivot on the ball of the right foot turning the heel in and move the body slightly to face the South West direction.

54d side view

**54d** Move your bodyweight over the right leg and step forward with the left leg facing the Southern direction and move forward with about 60% of weight over the left leg and 40% over the right leg. At the same time circle both arms down slightly to the right and push arms up and around to face the wind in coordination with the movement forward. Extend arms keeping elbows relaxed and arms rounded with hands slightly higher than shoulders. The He Gu (web of hand) of both hands are both facing each other and the hands are soft and relaxed.

## Face the wind to the left

54e          54e side view          54f

**54e** Keeping your shoulders and elbows relaxed, lift both arms in front of the body; the wrists are relaxed and the fingers are pointing to the ground. Bend the elbows and draw both hands back with the He Gu (web of hands) facing towards the Qi Hu (beneath collar bone). With your bodyweight on the right leg, pivot on the ball of the left foot turning the heel in and moving the body slightly to face the South East direction.

**54f** Move your bodyweight over the left leg and step forward with the right leg facing the Southern direction and move forward with about 60% of your weight over the right leg and 40% over the left leg. At the same time, circle both arms down slightly to the left and push arms up and around to face the wind in coordination with the movement forward. Extend your arms keeping the elbows relaxed and arms rounded with hands slightly higher than shoulders. The He Gu (web of hand) of both hands are facing each other and the hands are soft and relaxed.

Repeat face the wind left and right for a total of seven times finishing with your bodyweight forward over the right leg.

**Benefit:** These movements are beneficial to the Pancreas and can improve diabetes.

## 55. Stretching the arms on both sides 横膀

*In this movement Qi is dispersed when the hands push out and is nurtured when the movement pauses. This releases inner heat of the Lungs and stimulates the Heart, Small Intestine, Large Intestine and Lung Channels.*

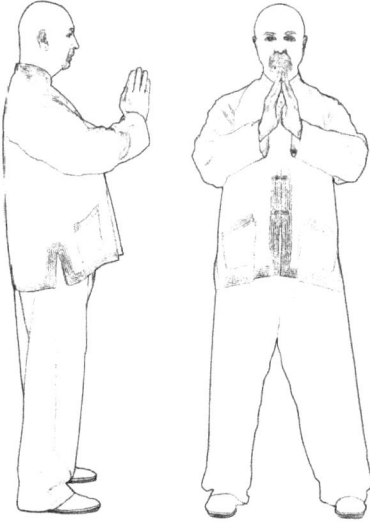

55a

55a side view

**55a** Keeping your bodyweight over the right leg, step up with the left leg placing the left foot parallel with the right foot and your bodyweight evenly distributed at about shoulder-width apart. Relax both arms and bring both palms together in front of the Middle Dan Tian (middle of chest between the nipples). The hands are soft and hollow in a devotional (prayer) position. Maintain this position for five seconds in meditation.

**55b** Swing both arms out and gently stretch the arms to both sides with the palms facing the Eastern and Western directions. Keep the shoulders and elbows relaxed, the palms facing outwards, the fingers pointing forward and the eyes looking straight ahead. Pause for two to three seconds.

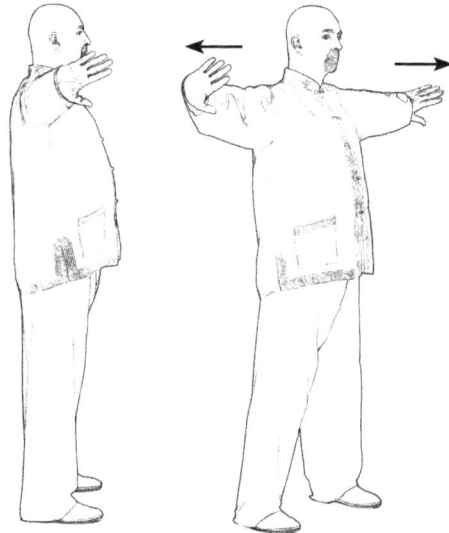

55b

55b diagonal view

## 56. Crossing the sea 过海

*These movements stimulate Qi into the Tai Yang (at the temple) and Lower Dan Tian (beneath the navel).*

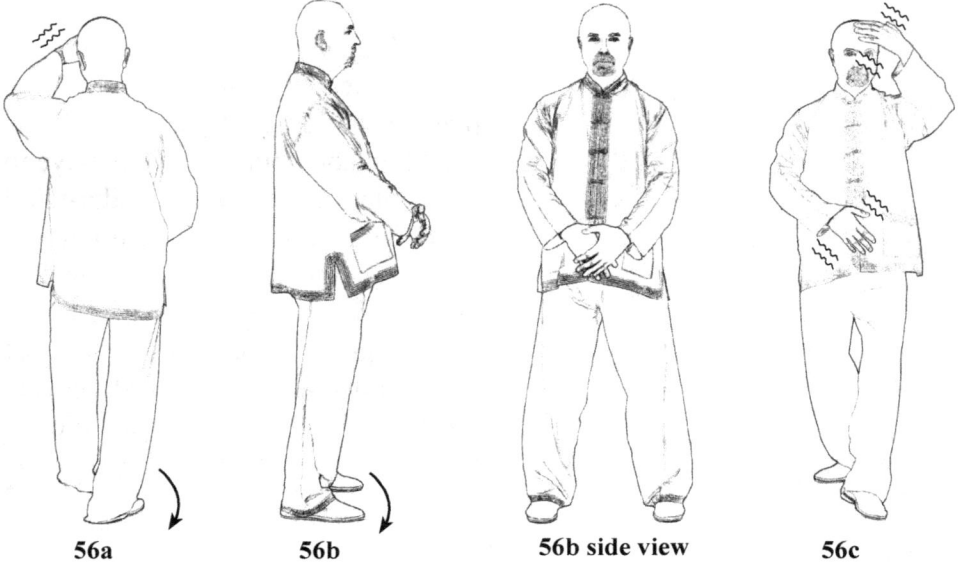

| 56a | 56b | 56b side view | 56c |

**56a** Turn the right toe in slightly and then move your bodyweight over the right leg. Pivot on the left heel and turn the whole body 90° to face the Eastern direction. Keep your bodyweight over the right leg with the left toes just touching the ground. The hands start to flutter and the right arm swings down with the Lao Gong (middle of palm) facing the Lower Dan Tian (area beneath the navel). The left arm swings up with the Lao Gong facing the Tai Yang (at the temple). The eyes are looking at the left hand sensing the Qi for three seconds.

**56b,c** Turn your body 180° to face the Western direction. Pivoting on the left heel hook the left toe in as far as feels comfortable, shift your bodyweight back onto the left leg and pivot on the right heel to turn the body to face the Western direction. Keep your bodyweight over the left leg and the right toes just touching the ground. At the same time, slowly change the position of the fluttering arms with the left Lao Gong (middle of palm) facing the Lower Dan Tian (area beneath the navel) and the right Lao Gong (middle of palm) facing the Tai Yang (at the temple). The eyes are looking at the right hand sensing the Qi for three seconds.

## 57. Flying over 飞荡

*This movement soothes the Qi through the Triple Heater (Sanjiao) and nurtures and disperses Qi.*

**Flying over to the west**

57a                         57b                         57c

**57a,b** Lower both fluttering arms to the side of the body with the palms facing up. Move your bodyweight forward over the right leg and lift the left heel off the ground. At the same time, swing both fluttering arms up in front of your body to about shoulder-height, keeping the shoulders and elbows relaxed and the fingers pointing to the ground.

**57c** Move your bodyweight back over the left leg and slightly lift the right toe as the fluttering arms pass by the hip area.

Repeat this forward and back rocking movement a total of three times with the right toe off the ground each time.

## Flying over to the east

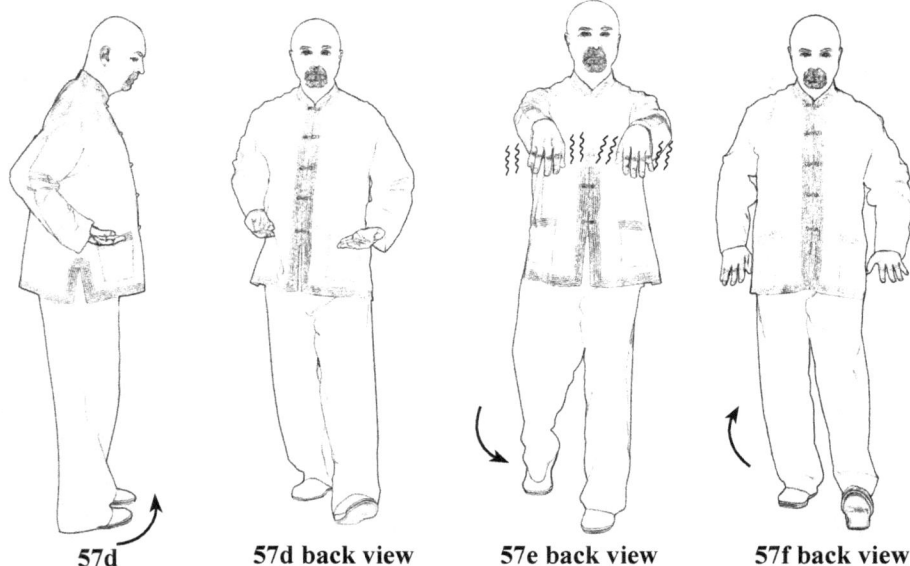

57d          57d back view        57e back view        57f back view

**57d** Pivoting on the right heel hook the right toe in as far as feels comfortable, shift your bodyweight back onto the right leg and pivoting on the left heel turn the body 180° to face the Eastern direction. The palms of both hands are facing up resting on the waist.

**57e** Move your bodyweight forward over the left leg and lift the right heel off the ground. At the same time, swing both fluttering arms up in front of your body to about shoulder-height, keeping the shoulders and elbows relaxed and the fingers pointing to the ground.

**57f** Move your bodyweight back onto the right leg as the fluttering arms pass by the hip area.

Repeat this forward and back rocking movement a total of three times with the left toe off the ground each time.

## 58.   Distribute the Qi and shaking 贯气颤动

*This movement nurtures and disperses Qi.*

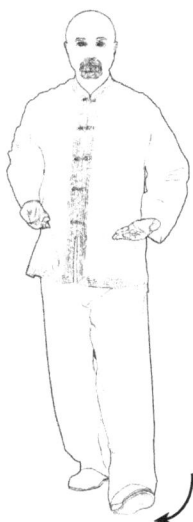 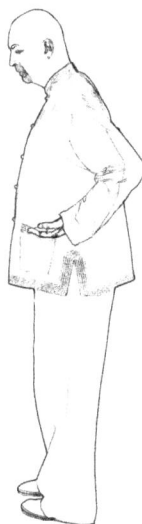

**58a back view**          **58b back view**

**58a**      Keeping your bodyweight over the right leg and pivoting on the left heel turn the left toe 90° to the right. Move your bodyweight back over the left leg and pivot on the right toe to turn the right heel in to the right.

**58b**      Both feet are parallel and your bodyweight is evenly distributed at about shoulder-width apart, facing the Southern direction. The palms of both hands are facing up and resting on the waist.

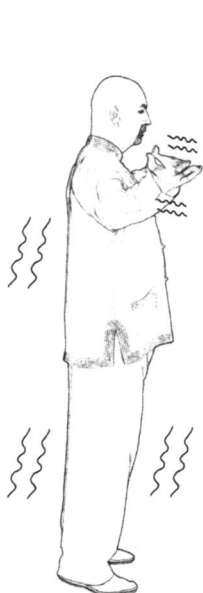

58c

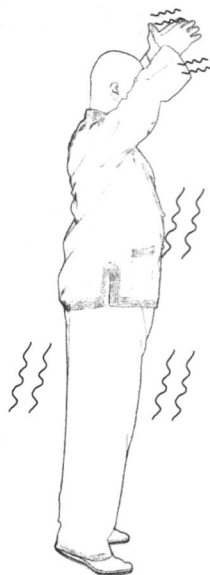

58d

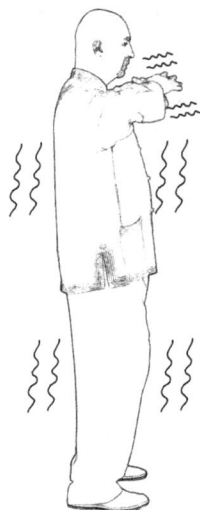

58e

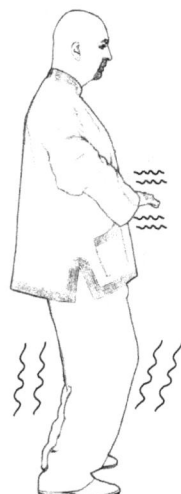

58f

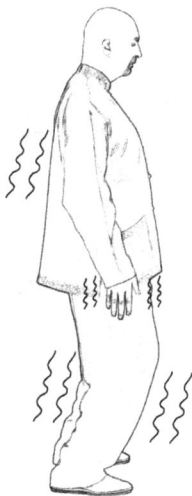

58g

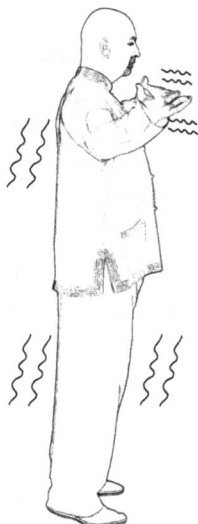

58h

**58c-h** Move your bodyweight to the balls of both feet and start to bounce up and down vibrating and shaking the whole body. At the same time, raise both fluttering arms up the side of the body with the palms face up, keeping your shoulders and elbows relaxed. Turn palms toward the Upper Dan Tian (between the eyebrows) and then lower fluttering arms down the front of the body distributing the Qi through the whole body.

Repeat for a total of seven times, bouncing on the balls of the feet and gently raising and lowering the knees in coordination with the fluttering arms; the whole body is vibrating and shaking.

**Benefit:** This movement dispels dampness from the body and aids arthritis and rheumatism and stimulates the Triple Heater (Sanjiao).

## 59. Vibrating the wings 抖翅

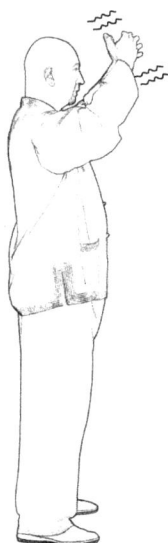 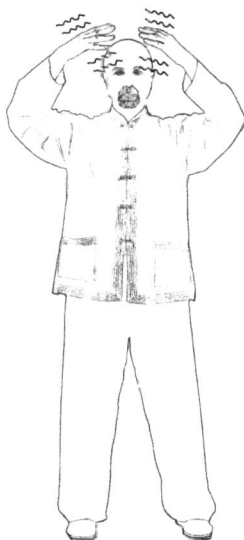 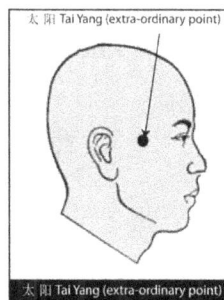

太 阳 Tai Yang (extra-ordinary point)

太 阳 Tai Yang (extra-ordinary point)

**59a**                                              **59a side view**

**59a** Slowly allow the vibrating and shaking to subside and lower both heels onto the ground and the arms to the side of the body. Raise your arms up over the head, keeping shoulders and elbows relaxed. Turn the Lao Gong (middle of palm) of both hands towards the Tai Yang (at the temple) and vibrate both hands at the temple three times, then pause. Repeat the vibrating of the wings two more times pausing for three seconds in between each one (a total of nine).

## 60. Looking down at the earth 俯瞰大地

*These movements regulate the Qi and stimulate the three Yin foot meridians (Kidney, Liver and Spleen). It also stimulates the Dai Mai Channel (around the waist).*

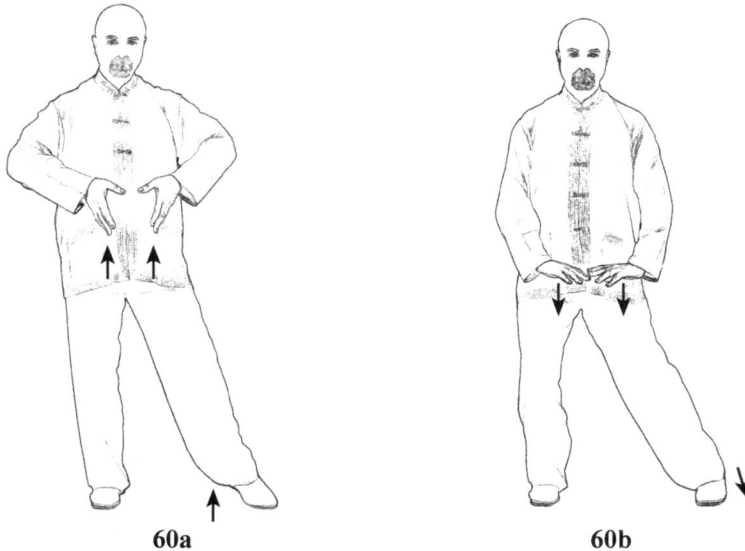

60a

60b

**60a,b** Move your bodyweight over the left leg and pivot on the ball of the right foot and turn the heel clockwise 90°. Move your bodyweight back over the right leg and step around with the left leg (hook step), placing the left foot parallel with the right foot facing the Western direction. At the same time, lower both arms and push down at the waist, keeping shoulders relaxed with the elbows bent and the arms rounded. The hands and fingers are soft and open with the He Gu (web of hand) facing each other. Coordinate the push down movement with moving your bodyweight over right leg, and then straightening the left leg pivot on the ball of the left foot pushing out the left heel to an angle of 45°. The eyes are looking straight ahead.

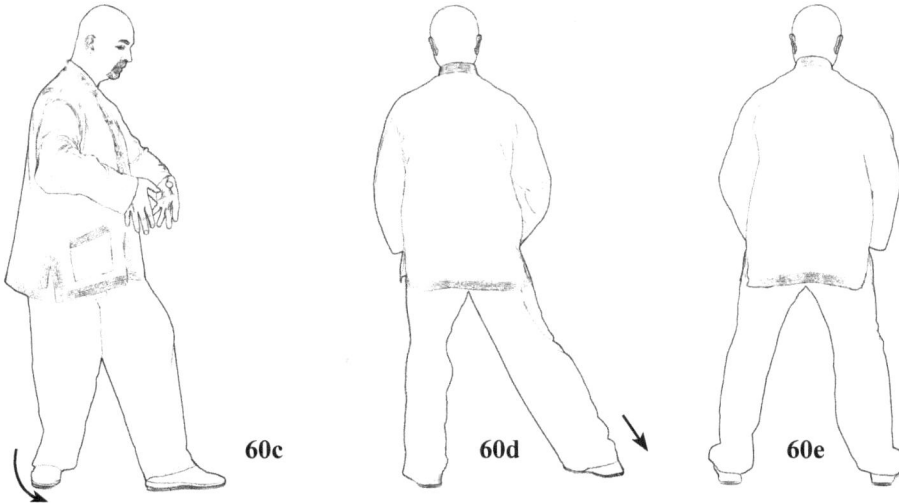

60c       60d       60e

**60c,d,e** Maintain your bodyweight over the right leg, relax hands and lift arms slightly with fingers pointing to the ground, at the same time pivot on the ball of the left foot and turn the heel counter clockwise as far as feels comfortable. Move your bodyweight back over the left leg and step around with the right leg (hook step), adjust feet so both are parallel facing the Eastern direction. Move bodyweight over left leg and straightening the right leg pivoting on the ball of the right foot pushing out the right heel to an angle of 45°. At the same time lower both arms and push down at the waist, keeping shoulders relaxed with the elbows bent and the arms rounded. The hands and fingers are soft and open with the He Gu (web of hand) of both hands facing each other. The eyes are looking straight ahead.

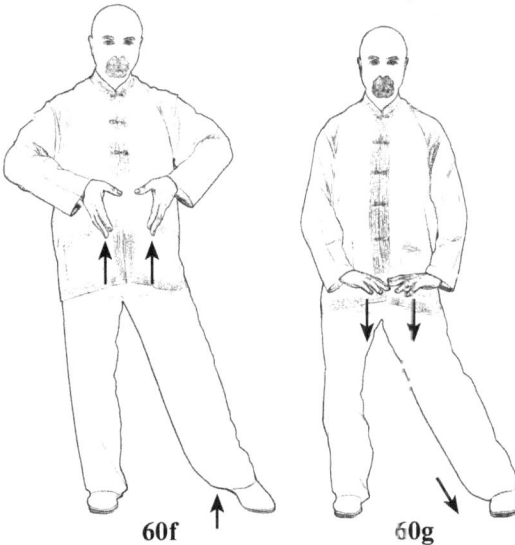

60f       60g

**60f,g** Maintain your bodyweight over the left leg; relax hands and lift arms slightly with fingers pointing to the ground, at the same time pivot on the ball of the right foot and turn the heel clockwise as far as feels comfortable. Move your bodyweight back over the right leg and step around with the left leg (hook step), adjust feet so both are parallel facing the Western direction. Move bodyweight over right leg and straightening the left leg pivot on the ball of the left foot pushing out the left heel to an angle of 45°. At the same time lower both arms and push down at the waist, keeping shoulders relaxed with the elbows bent and the arms rounded. The hands and fingers are soft and open with the He Gu (web of hand) facing each other. The eyes are looking straight ahead.

# 61. Raising the wings to watch the moon 抬膀迎月

*The circular movement of the hands receive good Qi to balance Yin and Yang energy.*

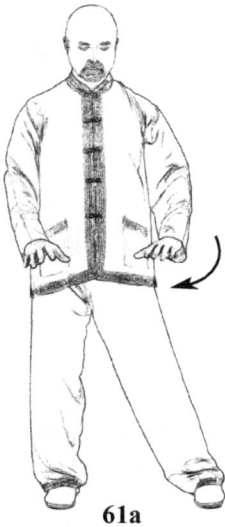

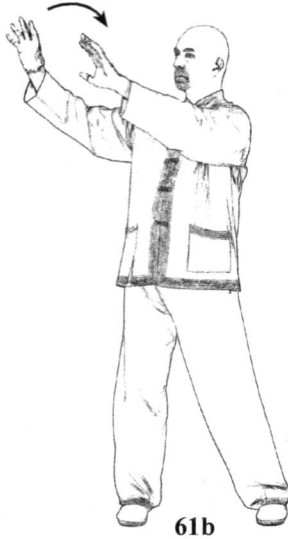

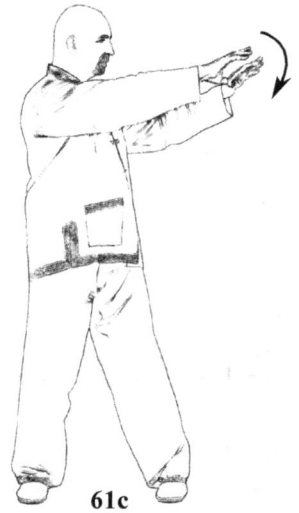

**61a**  **61b**  **61c**

**61a,b** Moving from the waist both arms swing to the left keeping shoulders relaxed and elbows slightly bent. The He Gu (web of hand) of both hands are facing each other and this is maintained through all the raising of the wings and watching the moon movements. Move 70% of your bodyweight over the left leg in coordination with the arms; both arms swing up and around in a circle to the right. Move your bodyweight in coordination with the arms finishing with about 70% of your bodyweight over the right leg.

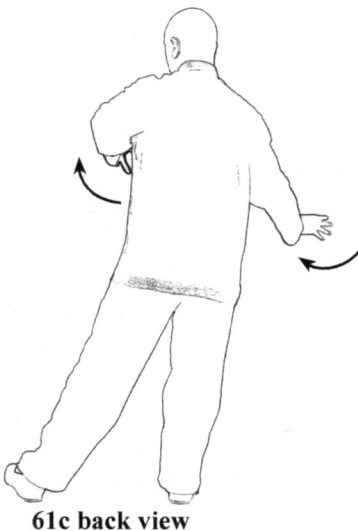

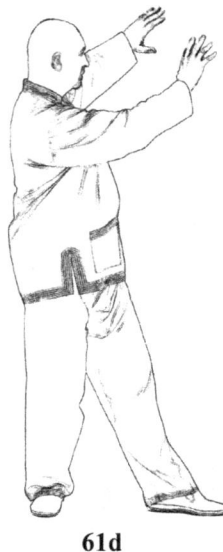

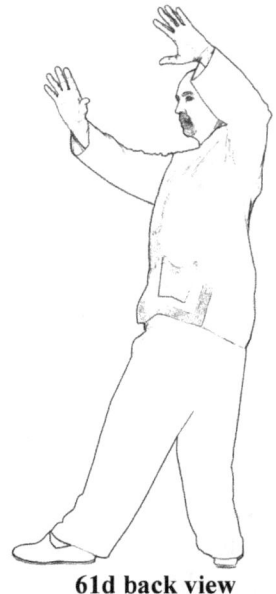

**61c back view**  **61d**  **61d back view**

**61c,d** Pivot on the ball of the left foot and turn the heel 90° counterclockwise; both arms circle around with the palms facing the South Eastern direction. The left hand is slightly higher in line with the head and the right hand is in line with the chest. Relax the right side of the body leaning slightly to the right and looking between the hands, watching the moon.

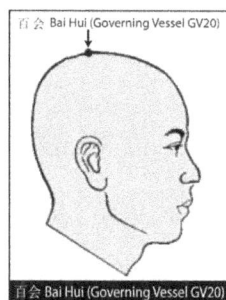

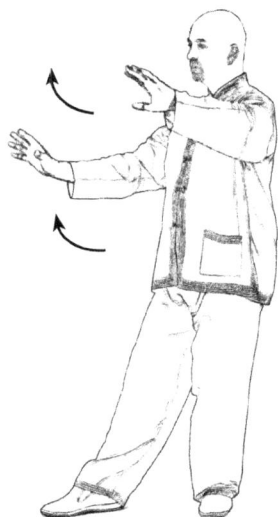

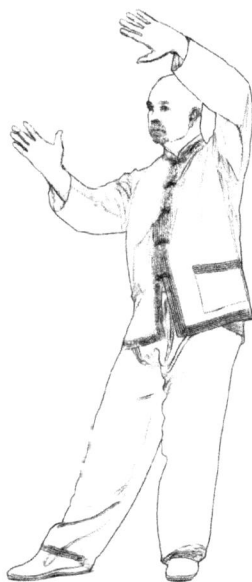

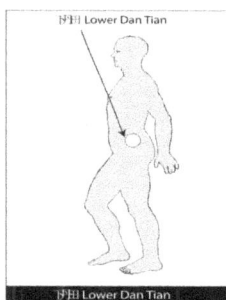

**61e**  **61f**

**61e-f** Gently straighten the body; the left hand drops slightly as the right hand rises keeping shoulders and elbows relaxed. Pivoting on the ball of the left foot turn the heel clockwise as far as feels comfortable. Move your bodyweight back over the left leg and pivot on the ball of the right foot, turning the body 180°. The arms move in coordination with the legs, the right hand above the head with the He Gu (web of hand) passing the Bai Hui at the top of the head and the left hand in front of the Lower Dan Tian (area beneath the navel). Circle both arms up and around with the left hand slightly higher and in line with the head and the right hand is in line with the chest with both palms facing the North West direction. Relax the right side of the body leaning slightly to the right and looking between the hands, watching the moon.

## 62. Rotating hands and chopping the Liver 大缠手

*In this movement, the circling of the hand around the top of the head eliminates inner heat by moving Qi from the top of the head to the soles of the feet. The chopping movement eliminates stale Qi from the Liver.*

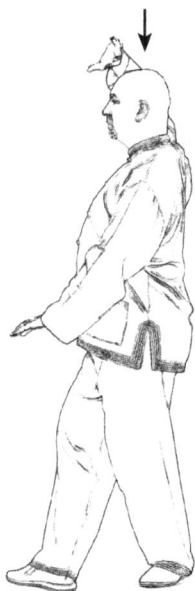

**62a**

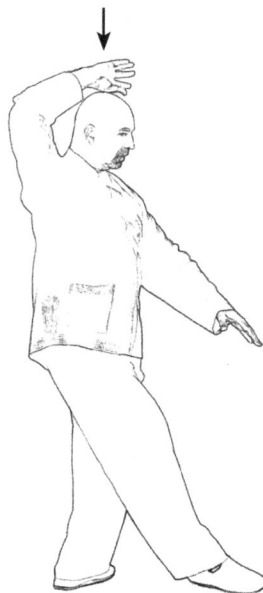

**62a back view**

**62a** Keep bodyweight over the left leg and gently straighten the body rotating the arms. The right hand is over the head with the He Gu (web of hand) passing the Bai Hui at the top of the head and the left hand is in front of the Lower Dan Tian (area beneath the navel). Pivoting on the ball of the right foot turn the heel clockwise as far as feels comfortable, step around with the left leg and place the left toe in front just touching the ground, facing the Northern direction. Both arms swing around with the body, the left Lao Gong (middle of palm) faces the Lower Dan Tian (area beneath the navel) and the right palm towards the waist.

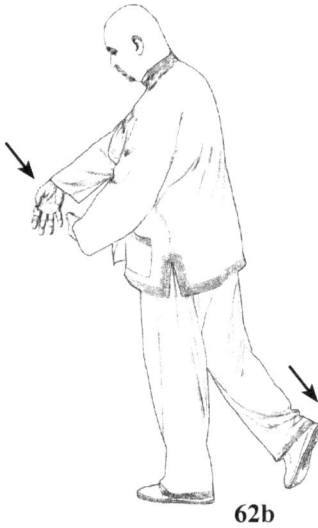

62b

62c

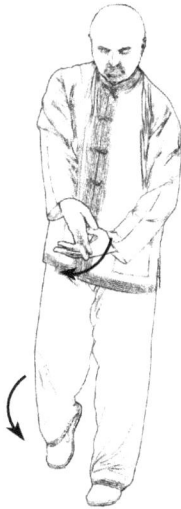

62b side view

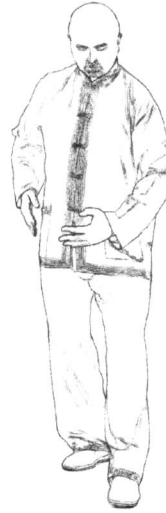

62cside view

**62b,c** Move your bodyweight forward over the left leg and lift the right heel. The right hand moves forward with the eyes looking at the right hand and gently touching the bottom of the left hand.

Circle the right hand on top of the left hand then quickly chop down the right side of the body to the waist, chopping the Liver. The eyes are looking at the left hand with the Lao Gong (middle of palm) facing the Lower Dan Tian (area beneath the navel). At same time quickly move your bodyweight back onto the right leg, making a sharp stomping and forceful movement grounding the weight onto the right heel. All your bodyweight is on the right leg with the left toe just touching the ground.

# 63. Flying up over the water 飘水飞上

*In this series of movements we are receiving the Qi by lifting the arms and the body, and dispersing the Qi when the arms and body are lowered.*

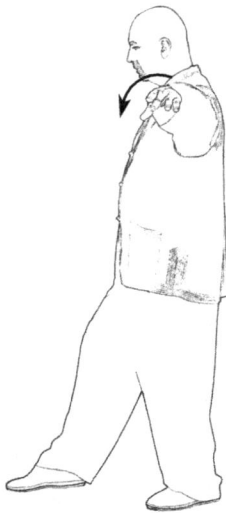
63a

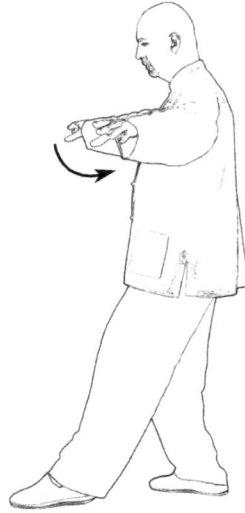
63b

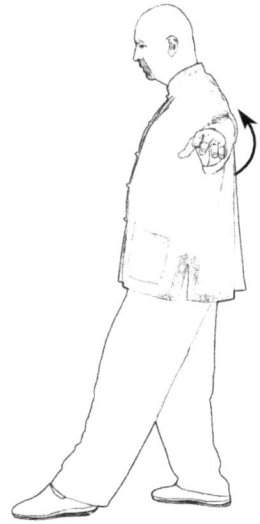
63c

**63a**  Move your bodyweight forward over the left leg and step up with the right leg with the right toes just touching the ground. Raise both arms to the side of the body, keep shoulders, elbows and wrists relaxed and the fingers pointing to the ground, lifting the wings.

**63b,c**  Relax the shoulders and drop both elbows, circling the arms behind and forward and then straighten the elbows by slightly pushing them out without locking them. This is a delicate movement. At the same time, tense the fingers slightly as the arms pass down and behind, then relax the hands as they straighten out. At the same time, bend the knees gently lowering and rising in coordination with the arms, the whole body moving together flying over the water. Repeat this bending and straightening three times. Step forward with left toe just touching the ground and repeat three flying movements. Then step forward again with right toe just touching the ground and repeat three arm movements together with three leg movements, the total of 'Flying over the Water' is nine times.

## 64. Holding and gathering the Qi 三抱收气

*Movement 64 is the strongest movement for these benefits. The Qi comes through the Middle Dan Tian (middle of chest between the nipples) and as we draw the arms back the Qi is gathered and stored in the Lower Dan Tian (beneath the navel).*

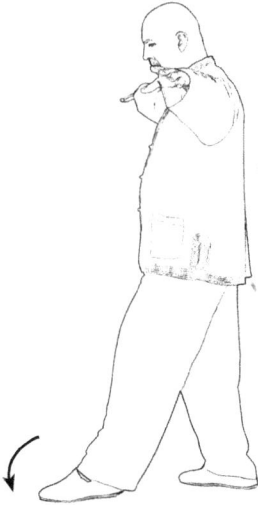 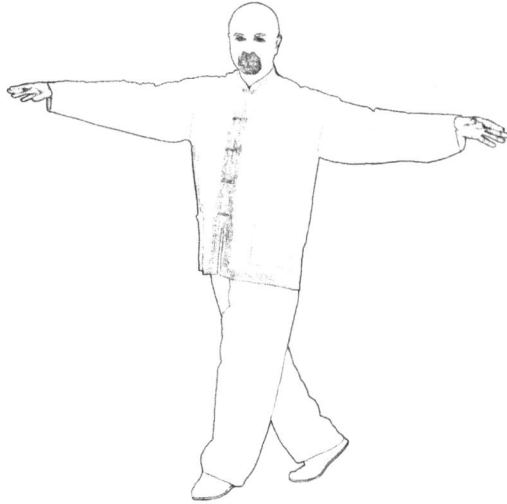

**64a**                                    **64b**

**64a** Move your bodyweight forward over the right leg and step forward with the left leg with the toes just touching the earth.

**64b** Lift the left toe and turn the foot 90° counter-clockwise. Twist the body turning 90° from the waist to face the Western direction. Step around with the right leg so that the right foot is parallel with the left foot at about shoulder-width apart. Both arms are out to the side with palms facing the ground.

**64c**                     **64d**                    **64e**                    **64f**

**64c**  Move your bodyweight over the right leg and step in closer with the left toe just touching the ground. The left arm scoops under the right arm, like holding a large ball of Qi. The Lao Gong (middle of palm) of both hands are facing each other.

**64d,e**  Step back with the left leg to about shoulder-width apart and transfer your weight back onto the left leg. The right and left arm sweep back in coordination with the backward movement, gathering the Qi to the Lower Dan Tian (area beneath the navel). The right hand passes around the inside and circles the left hand.

**64f**  Move your bodyweight forward over the right leg. The Lao Gong (middle of palm) of the right hand faces the left Qi Hu (beneath collar bone) with the eyes looking at the hand. The fingers of the left hand are touching the Dai Mai (below the ribs) at the left waist with the shoulders and elbow relaxed in a circle resting on the waist.

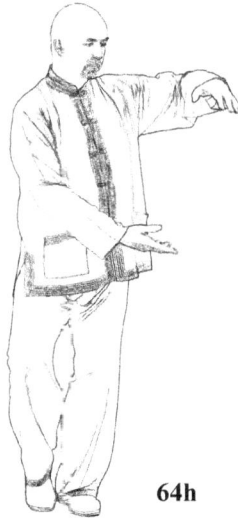

**64g** 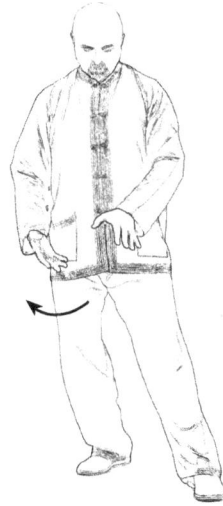 **64h** 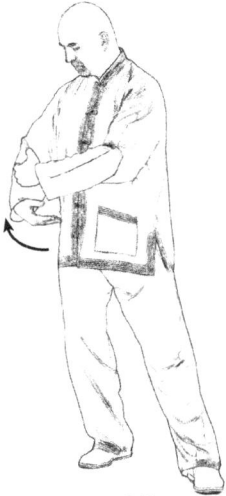 **64i**

**64g,h** Move your bodyweight over the left leg and step back with the right leg closer with the right toe just touching the ground. The right hand sweeps underneath as the left hand scoops over the top. The Lao Gong (middle of palm) of both hands are facing each other holding the Qi.

**64j** 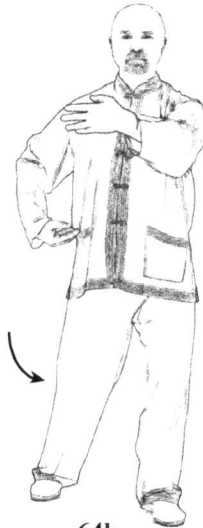 **64k**

**64i,j** Step back with the right leg to about shoulder-width apart and transfer your weight back onto the right leg. The left and right arm sweep back in coordination with the backward movement gathering Qi to the Lower Dan Tian (area beneath the navel). The left hand passes around the inside and circles the right hand.

**64k** Move your bodyweight forward over the left leg. The Lao Gong (middle of palm) of the left hand faces the right Qi Hu (beneath collar bone) with the eyes looking at the hand. The fingers of the right hand are touching the Dai Mai (below the ribs) at the right waist with the shoulder and elbow relaxed in a circle.

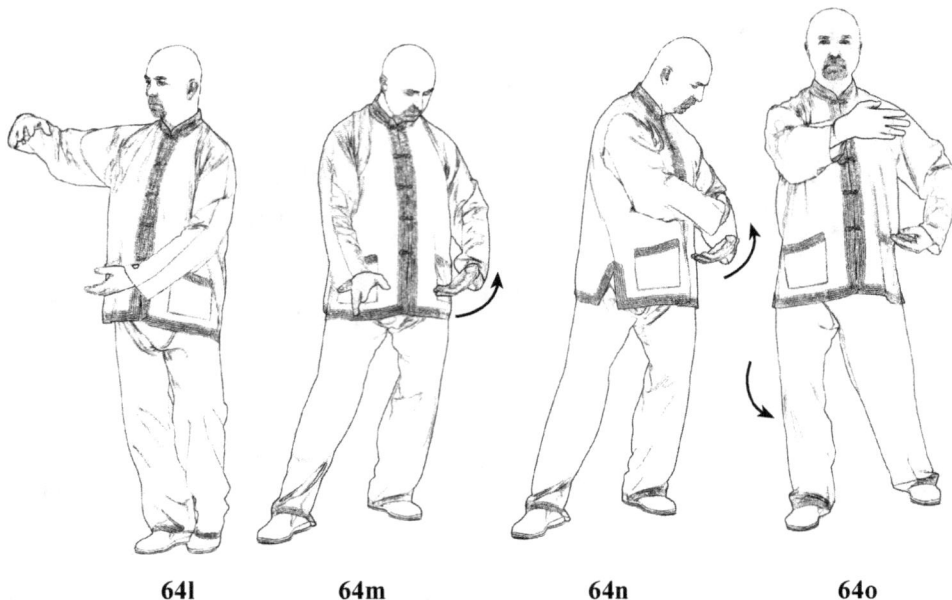

| 64l | 64m | 64n | 64o |

**64l,m** Move your bodyweight over the right leg and step in closer with the left toe just touching the ground. The left arm scoops under the right arm, like holding a large ball. The Lao Gong (middle of palm) of both hands are facing each other holding the Qi.

**64n** Step back with the left leg to about shoulder-width apart and transfer the weight back onto the left leg. The right and left arm sweep back in coordination with the backward movement, gathering the Qi to the Lower Dan Tian (area beneath the navel). The right hand passes around the inside and circles the left hand.

**64o** Move your bodyweight forward over the right leg. The Lao Gong (middle of palm) is facing the left Qi Hu (beneath collar bone) with the eyes looking at the hand. The fingers of the left hand are touching the Dai Mai (below the ribs) at the left waist with the shoulder and elbow relaxed in a circle.

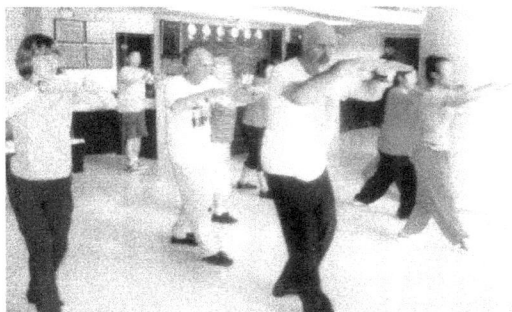

**Facing the wind and flying up** 看 风 上 飞

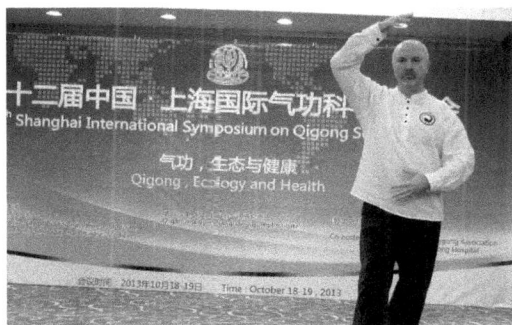

**Crossing the sea** 过 海

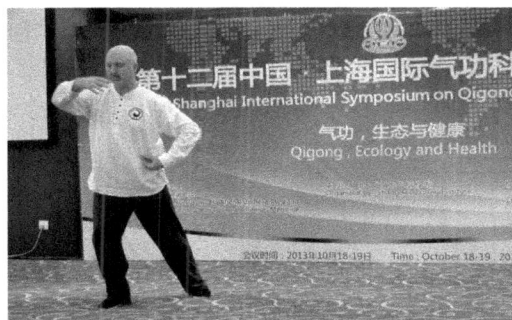

**Holding and gathering the Qi** 三 抱 收 气

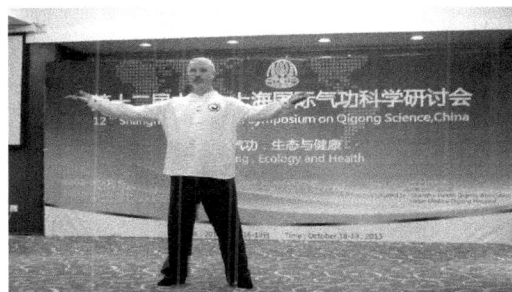

**Close** 收 式

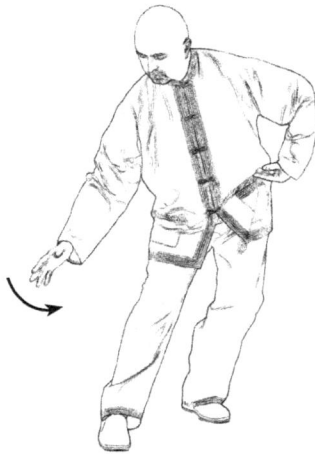

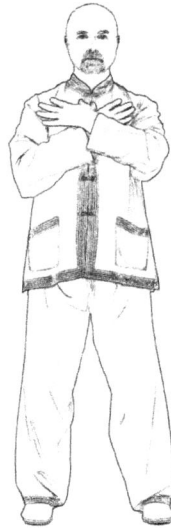

**64p**                                    **64q**

**64p,q** Move your bodyweight back onto the left leg bending slightly forward from the waist. The right arm scoops forward lifting up the right leg. Gently straighten the back and step back with the right leg placing the right foot parallel with the left foot. The right arm sweeps up with the Lao Gong (middle of palm) over the left Qi Hu (beneath collar bone) and the left arms sweeps up crossing the right arm with the left Lao Gong over the right Qi Hu (beneath collar bone).

**Benefit:** Movements 54 to 64 improve the function of the heart and lungs and help with bronchitis and asthma.

# Close 收式

a

b

c

d

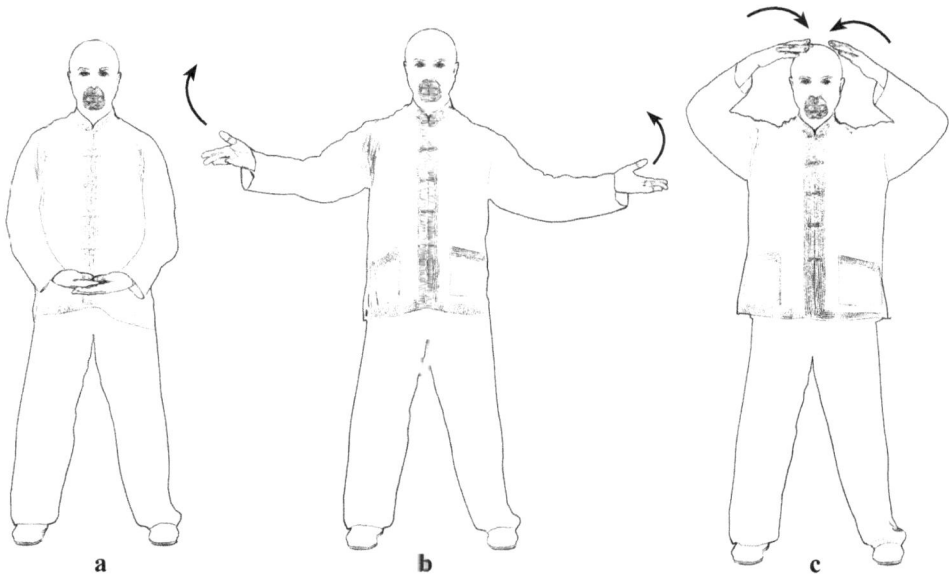

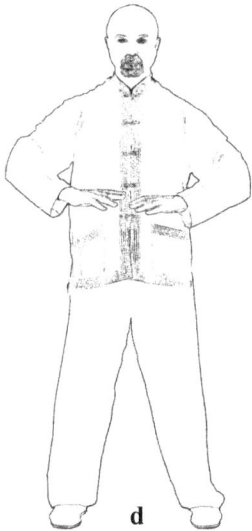

**a**  Slowly lower both arms in front of the body with the left palm resting on the right palm in front of the abdomen.

**b,c,d**  Lift your arms up overhead keeping the shoulders relaxed, and guide Qi to the top of the head, to the chest and to the Lower Dan Tian (area beneath the navel). Repeat a total of three times.

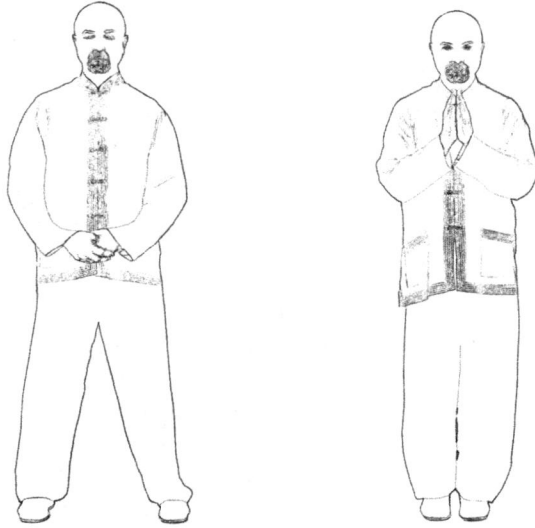

The tip of your right thumb touches the left Lao Gong (middle of palm), relaxing hands and fingers. Hands make a Yin Yang shape (Taiji). Place hands over the Lower Dan Tian (area beneath the navel). Close the eyes in meditation.

# Close with meditation

After practising the dynamic moving sections of the Da Yan Wild Goose Qigong, we practise the static or stillness section. This part of our practice is very important; when the body comes to a complete stop, the Qi keeps moving and through the tranquillity of the mind, the Qi will come into order. It's what we call the 'processing' stage; it's important to keep your thinking mind out of the way and to allow the Qi to do its work.

The final stage is ideally fifteen minutes of meditation, either sitting cross-legged on the floor or on the edge of a chair keeping the back straight. The chin is tucked in, with the tip of the tongue on the top palate of the mouth, just behind the teeth. Breathe naturally in and out through the nose. Sensing the breath and sensing the peace. Allow the breath to become smooth and even and the mind to rest for at least five minutes. Turn the hands in over the Dan Tian, the area beneath the navel, with one hand on top of the other. Allow your mind, breath and energy to settle. When breathing in, the abdomen gently pushes out into your hands. When breathing out gently push the hands in. Relax and feel the whole body breathe for another five minutes. After the face rubbing routine (on the next page), place the hands with palms down on the knees sensing the inner peace. Through the peace, allow the heart to open like a smile, with a wave of loving kindness permeating from the heart through the whole body. Just relax and let it go out through every cell. Every cell of the body is smiling with the radiance of the universe as you become one with the universe for another five minutes.

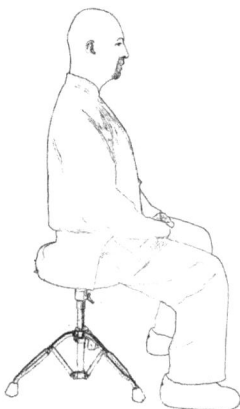

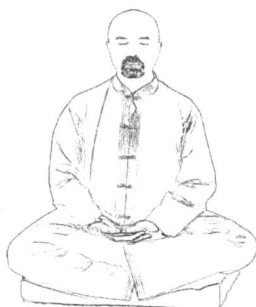

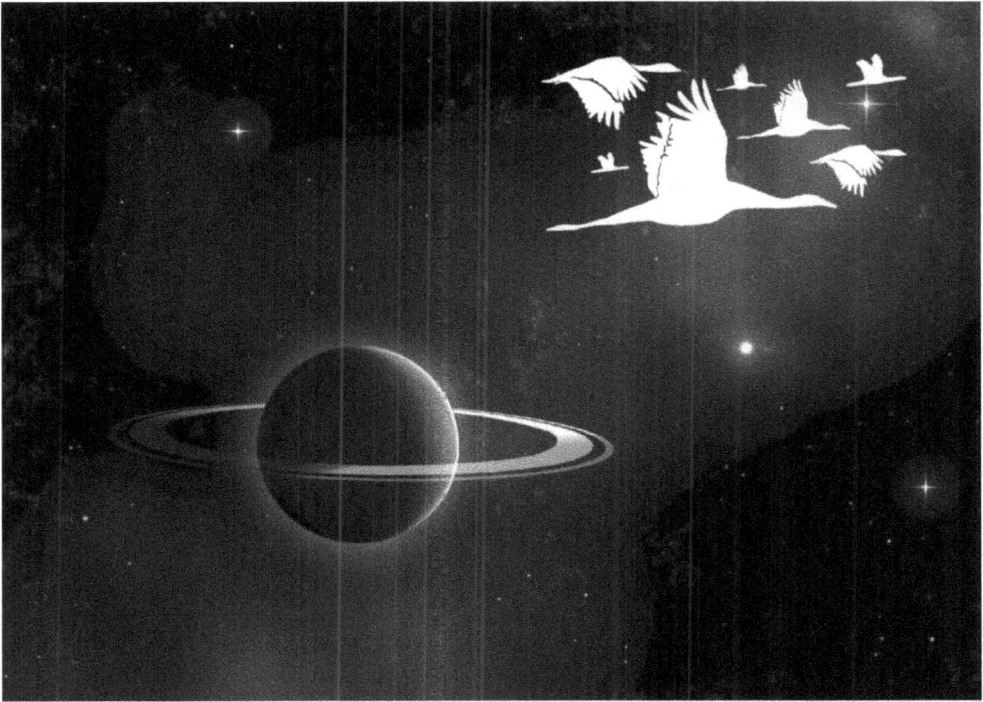

# Chapter 7
# Gathering the Qi and Rubbing the Face

Da Yan - Wild Goose Qigong
The 2nd 64 movements

# Gathering the Qi and Rubbing the Face

The practice of Qigong helps clear the energy channels and dredges the meridians of stagnant Qi. This allows the Qi to flow smoothly through the body and creates an energy or Qi field.

We generally feel this Qi field in the hands. To gather and refine the Qi move the hands in and out as follows:

## Gathering the Qi

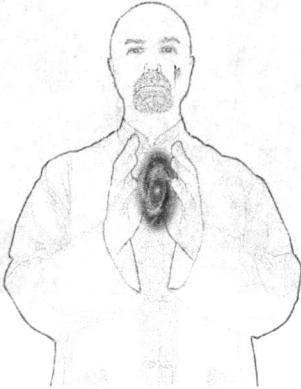

**A**

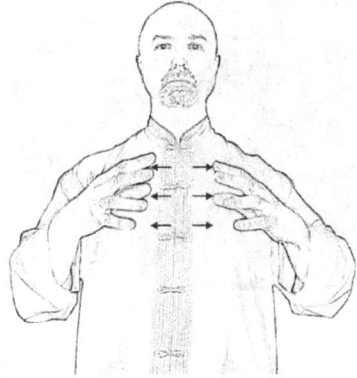

**B**

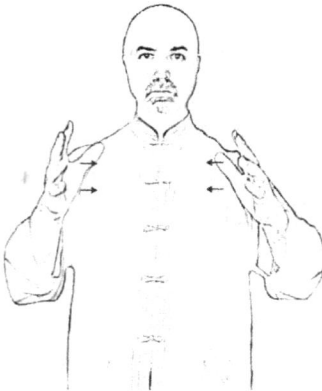

**C**

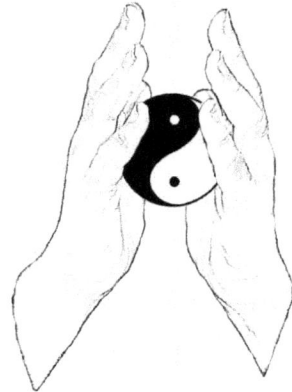

**D**

**A** Hold the hands in front of the body at chest height as if holding a ball of energy or light.

**B** Slightly draw the hands away from each other tensing the fingers.

**C** Then push the hands closer compressing the Qi between the hands.

**Repeat six times.**

**D** Relax and feel. We will generally feel warmth, like a field of energy between the hands. This creates a polarity as the left hand is Yang (positive) and the right hand is Yin (negative).

Now that the hands are charged with Qi it's a time for healing by placing the hands on a sore or injured part of your body or by massaging the face. Your face has many meridian acupuncture points that connect the meridians to the internal organs.

## Face rubbing

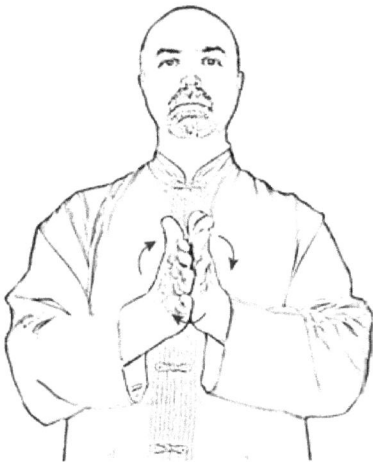

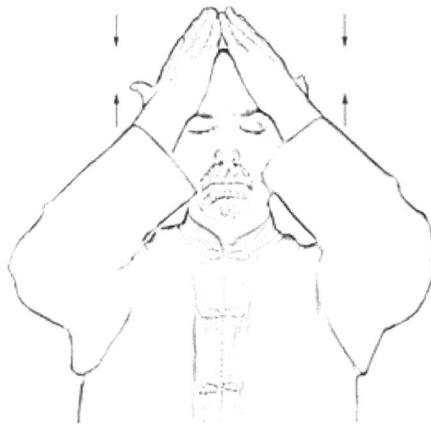

| A | B |

**A** Rub the hands together and bring the healing energy through your heart into your hands.

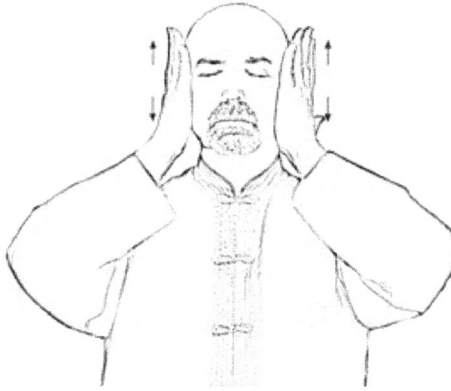

C

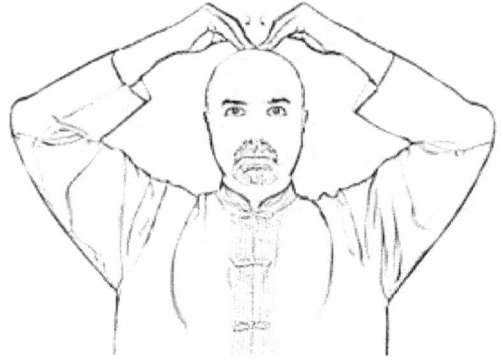

D

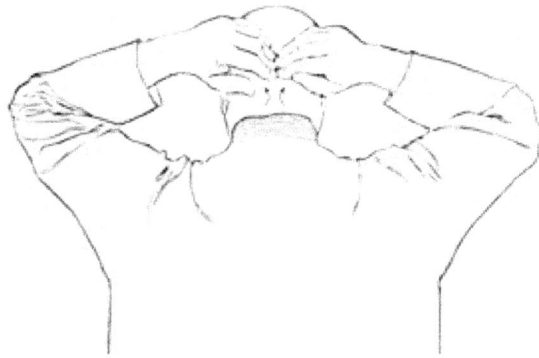

E

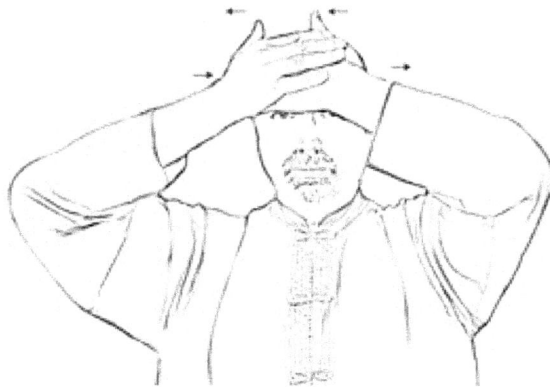

F

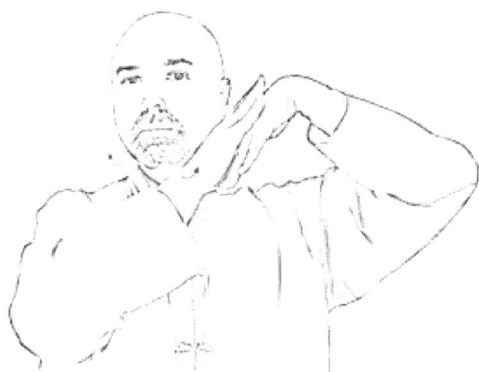

**G**

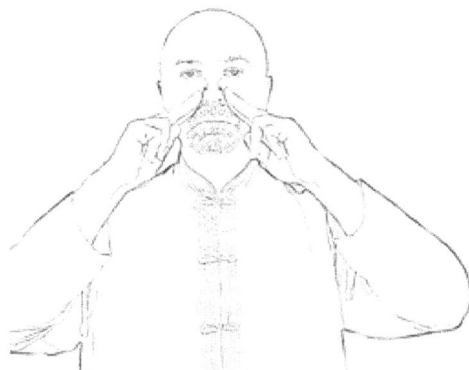

**H**

**B, C**  Place the warm palms over your eyes (liver). Feel the warmth going in. Then rub the hands up and down from the forehead to the chin, the side of the face, then around the eyes and cheeks in a circular motion, like washing the face.

Rub around the ears with the tip of the fingers massaging around the outside of the ears down to the ear lobe. With the tips of the fingers, massage around the inside of the ear following all the grooves, stimulating the kidneys.

**D, E**  With the tips of the fingers, massage back through the hair and then rub the back of the neck. Gently massage the base of the skull, the top of the head and massage up over the head and scalp.

**F, G,**  With one hand on top of the other rub the palm across the
**H**      forehead and then rub around the chin letting the knuckles massage the jaw. Rub the fingers down the sides of the nose and around the cheek bones (lung).

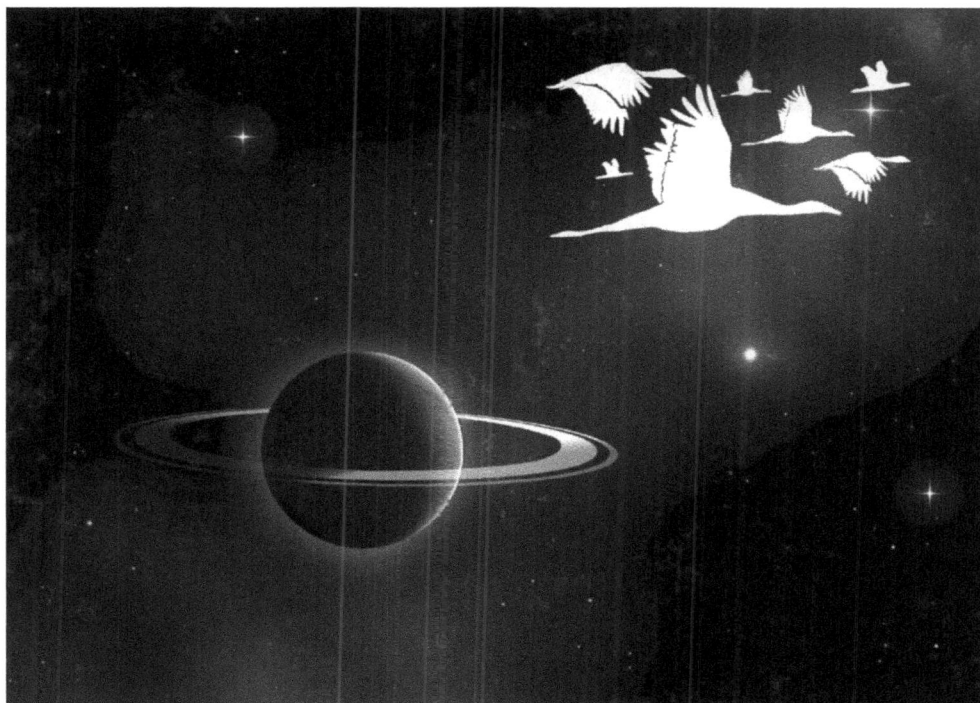

# Chapter 8
# Meridian Charts

Da Yan - Wild Goose Qigong
The 2nd 64 movements

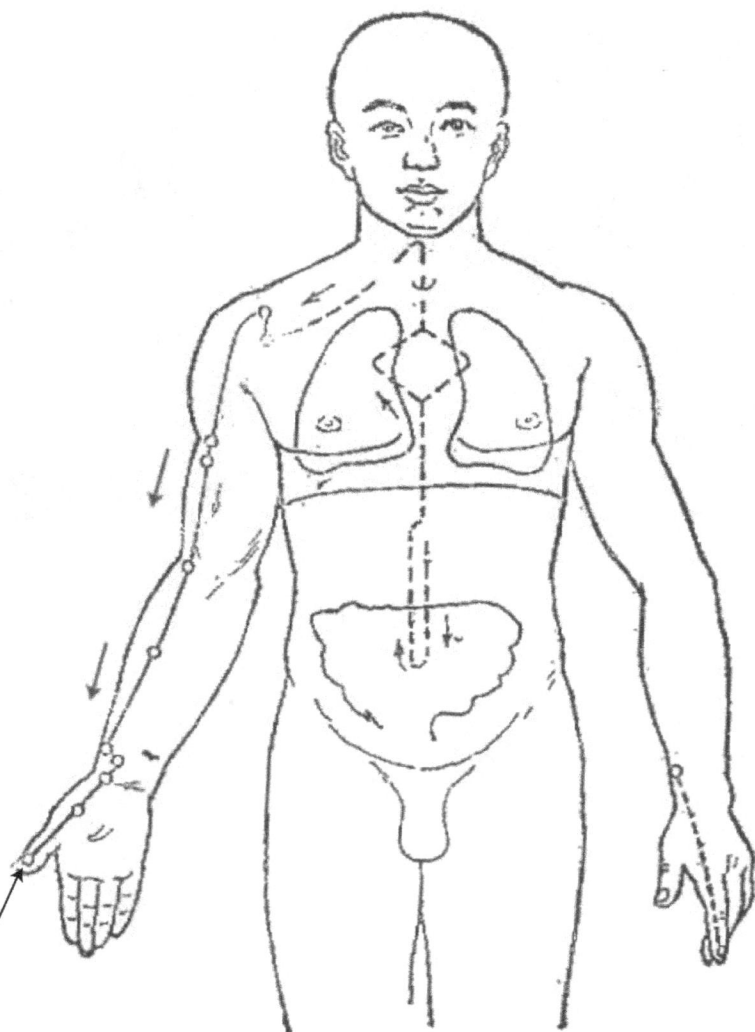

# 肺经 Lung Channel

少商  Shao Shang
(Lung LU11)

# 大肠经 Large Intestine Meridian

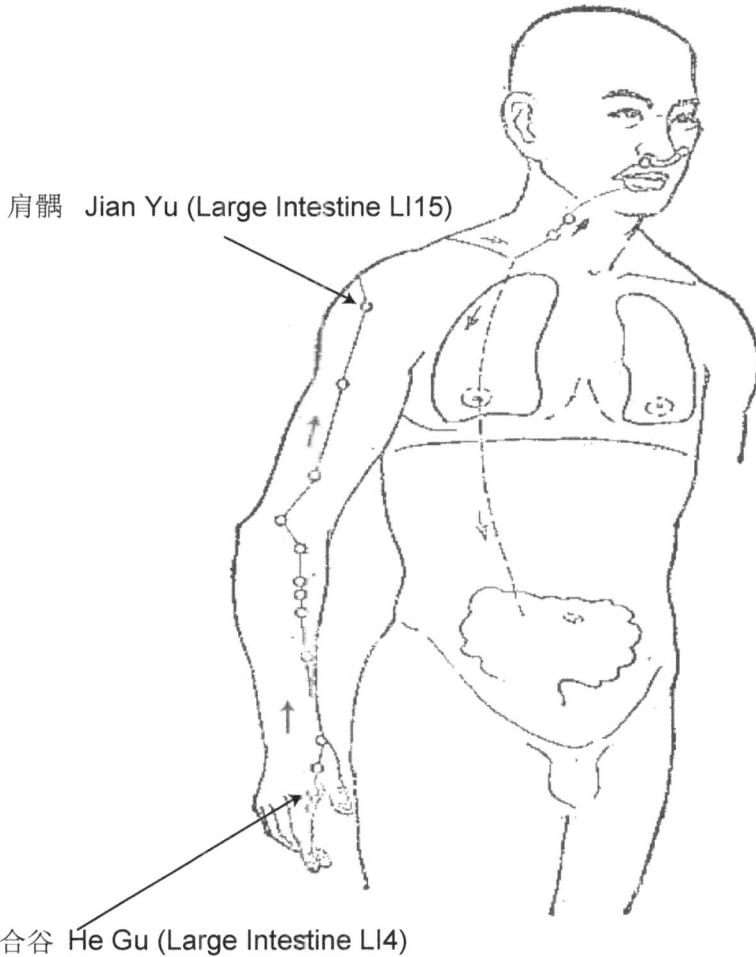

肩髃 Jian Yu (Large Intestine LI15)

合谷 He Gu (Large Intestine LI4)

No 2. The Large Intestine Meridian (Yang) originates from the outside of the index finger through the He Gu, along the outside of the arm to the shoulder, to the neck and finishes on the opposite side of the face near the nose and cheek bone.

# 脾经 Spleen Meridian

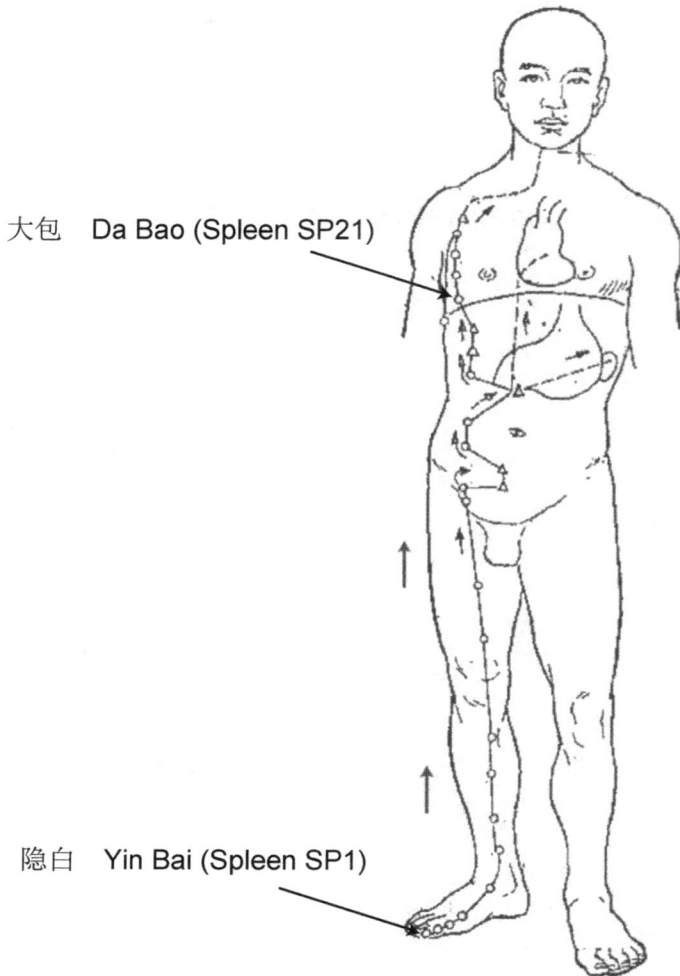

大包　Da Bao (Spleen SP21)

隐白　Yin Bai (Spleen SP1)

No 3. The Spleen Meridian (Yin) originates from the outside of the big toe, and rises up past the ankle the inside of the leg to the hip, through the abdomen to the chest and up to the oesophagus and under the tongue.

# 胃经 Stomach Meridian

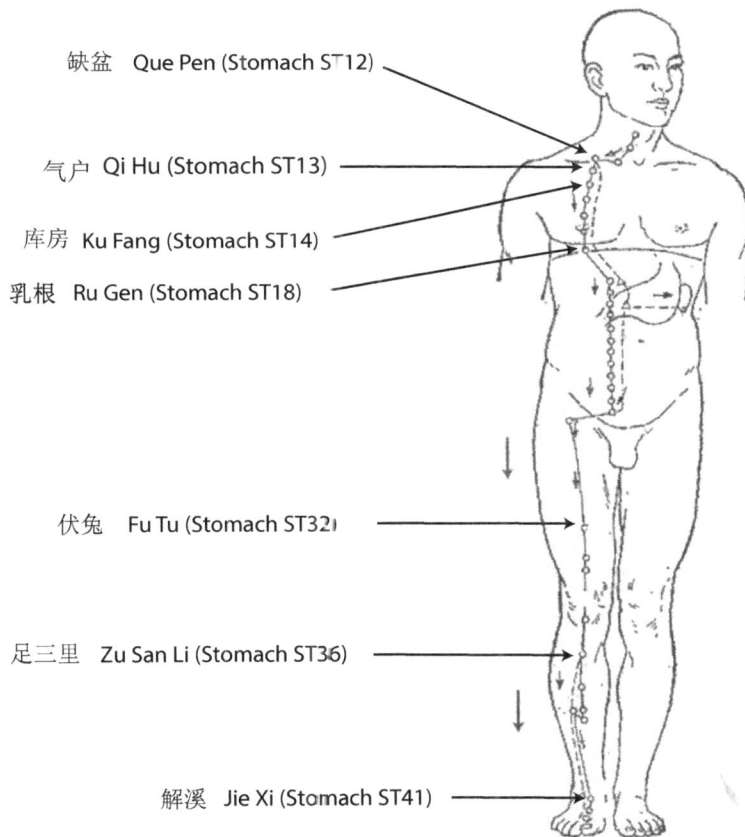

缺盆　Que Pen (Stomach ST12)

气户　Qi Hu (Stomach ST13)

库房　Ku Fang (Stomach ST14)

乳根　Ru Gen (Stomach ST18)

伏兔　Fu Tu (Stomach ST32)

足三里　Zu San Li (Stomach ST36)

解溪　Jie Xi (Stomach ST41)

No 4. The Stomach Meridian (Yang) originates from beneath the eye, down to the corner of the mouth, around the jaw, down the neck to the nipple, and down the body to the pubic bone. It then continues down the front of the leg to the front of the ankle and finishes on the outside of the second toe.

# 肝经 Liver Meridian

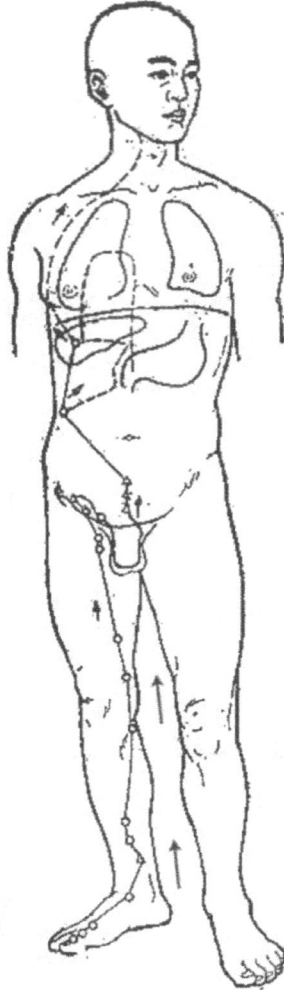

No 5. The Liver Meridian (Yin) originates from the inside of the big toe, rises up the inside of the leg into the body past the hip, and finishes at the lower rib area.

# 胆经 Gall Bladder Meridian

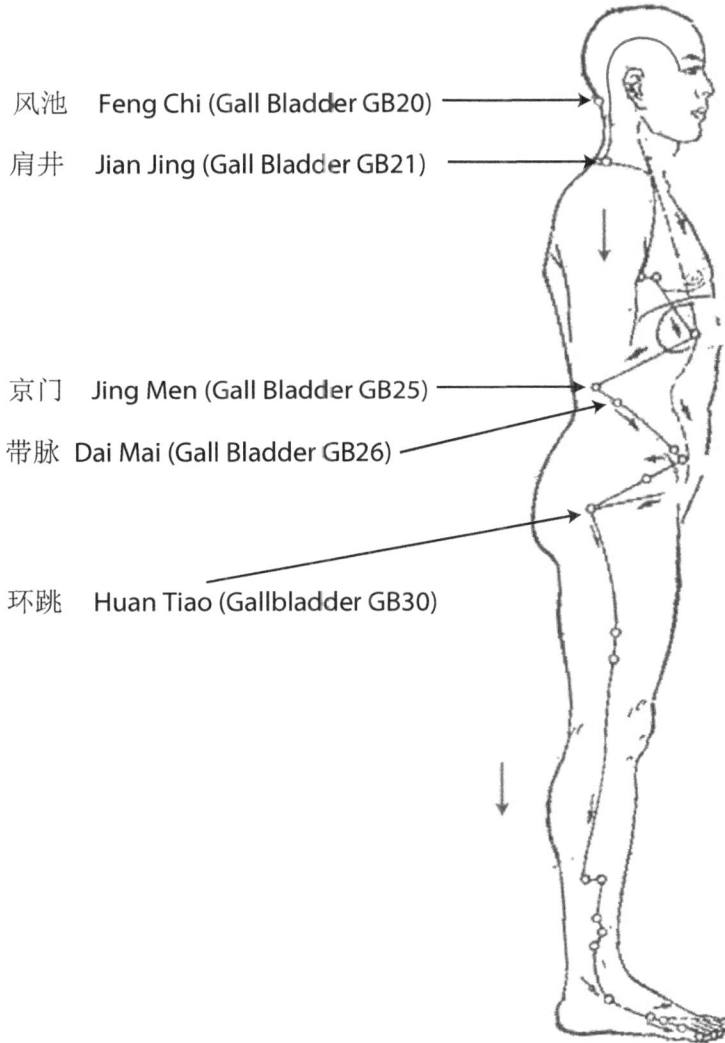

风池　Feng Chi (Gall Bladder GB20) ⟶

肩井　Jian Jing (Gall Bladder GB21) ⟶

京门　Jing Men (Gall Bladder GB25) ⟶

带脉　Dai Mai (Gall Bladder GB26) ⟶

环跳　Huan Tiao (Gallbladder GB30)

No 6. The Gall Bladder Meridian (Yang) originates from the outer corner of the eye, runs around the ear, down the neck, under the arm and down the side of the body, the outside of the leg, the outside of the foot and finishes at the outside of the fourth toe.

# 肾经 Kidney Meridian

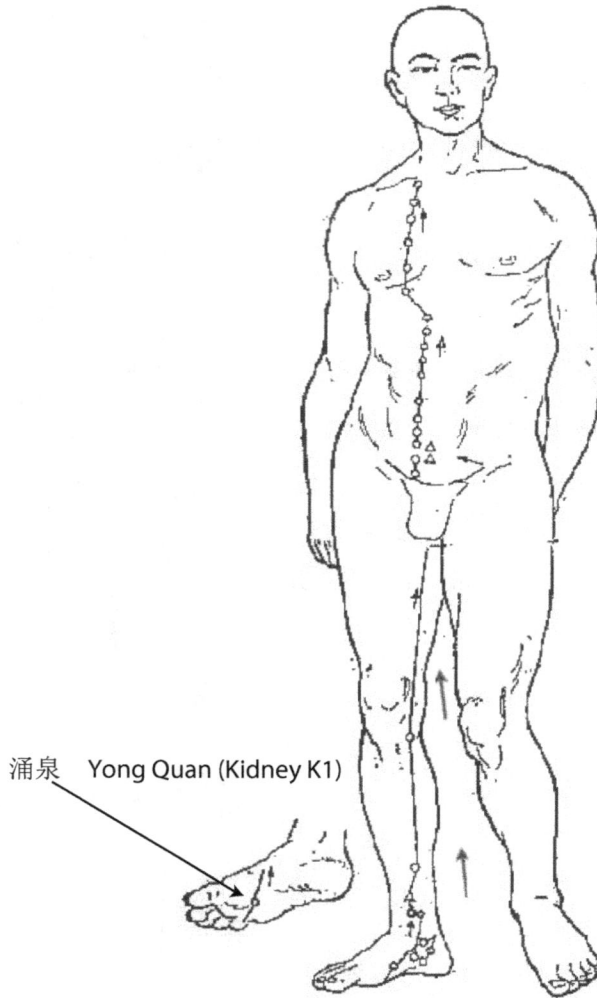

涌泉    Yong Quan (Kidney K1)

No 7. The Kidney Meridian (Yin) originates from the sole of the foot and rises up the inside of the leg, through the abdomen to the collar bone.

# 膀胱经 Urinary Bladder Meridian

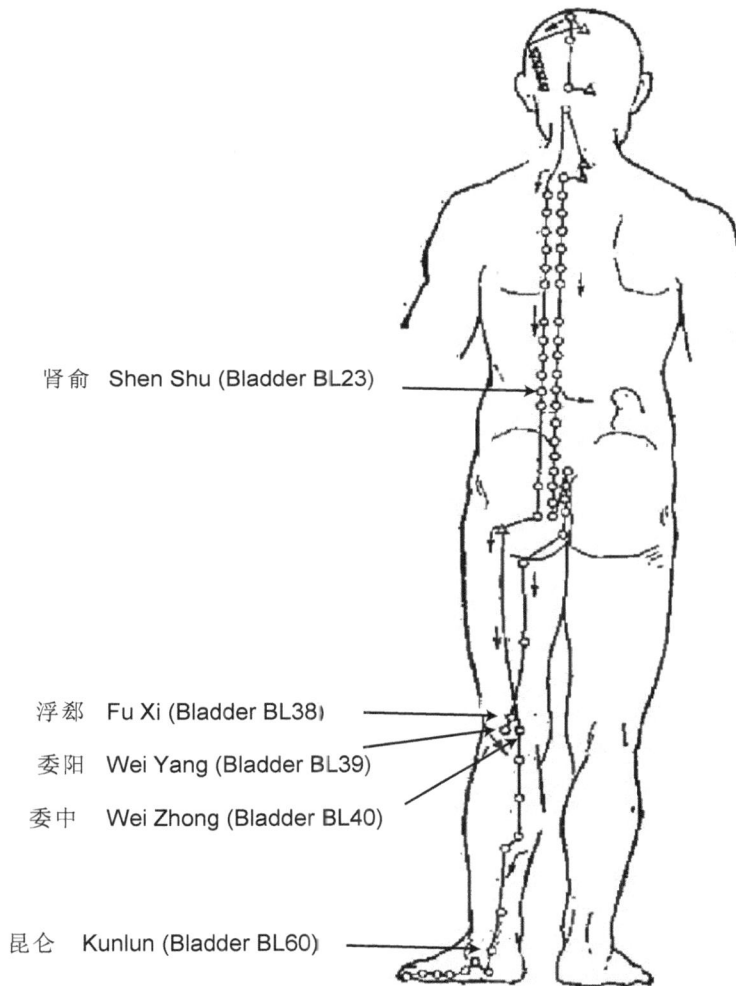

肾俞 Shen Shu (Bladder BL23)

浮郄 Fu Xi (Bladder BL38)

委阳 Wei Yang (Bladder BL39)

委中 Wei Zhong (Bladder BL40)

昆仑 Kunlun (Bladder BL60)

No 8. The Bladder Meridian (Yang) originates near the eyebrow and goes back over the head, down the back to the hip, the back of the legs to the heel, then along the outside of the foot finishing on the outside of the small toe.

# 心 经 Heart Meridian

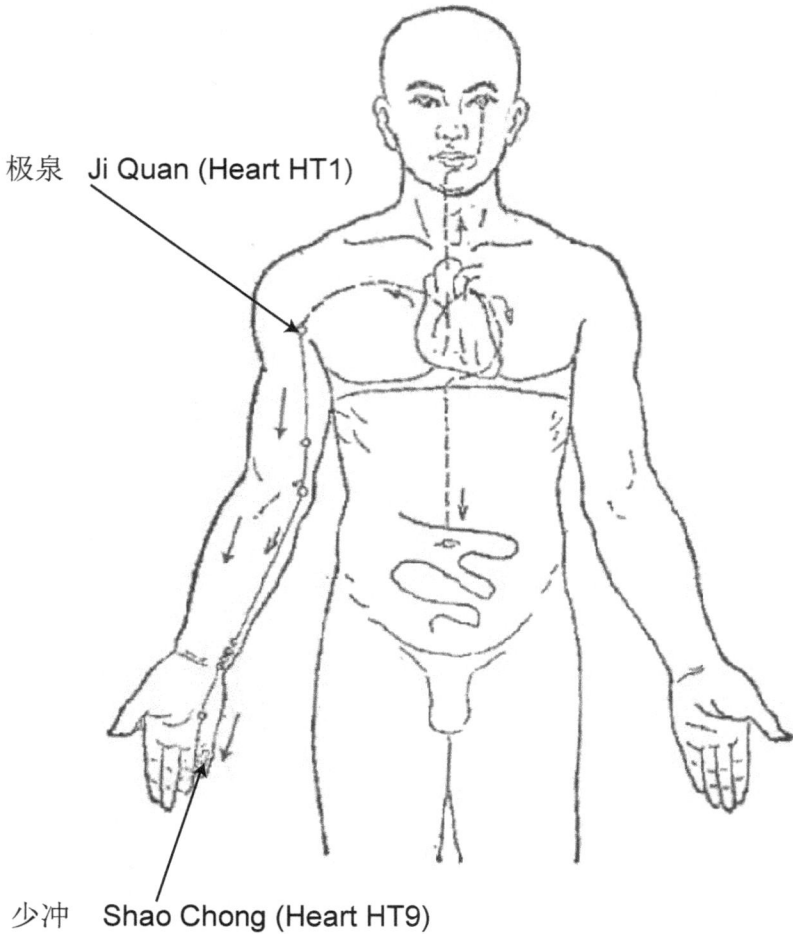

极泉　Ji Quan (Heart HT1)

少冲　Shao Chong (Heart HT9)

No 9. The Heart Meridian (Yin) originates from the armpit, past the elbow to the outside of the wrist finishing at the end of the inside of the small finger.

# 小肠经 Small Intestine Meridian

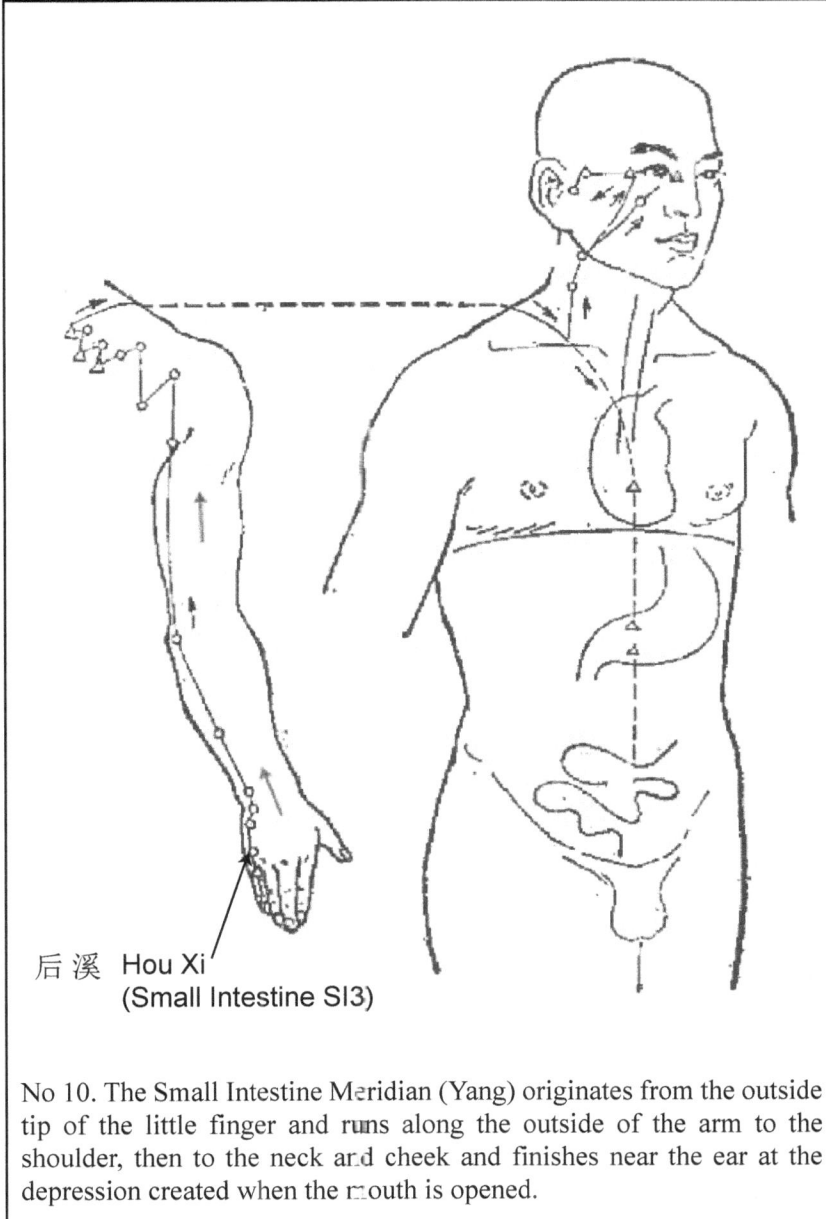

后溪 Hou Xi
(Small Intestine SI3)

No 10. The Small Intestine Meridian (Yang) originates from the outside tip of the little finger and runs along the outside of the arm to the shoulder, then to the neck and cheek and finishes near the ear at the depression created when the mouth is opened.

# 心包经 Pericardium Meridian

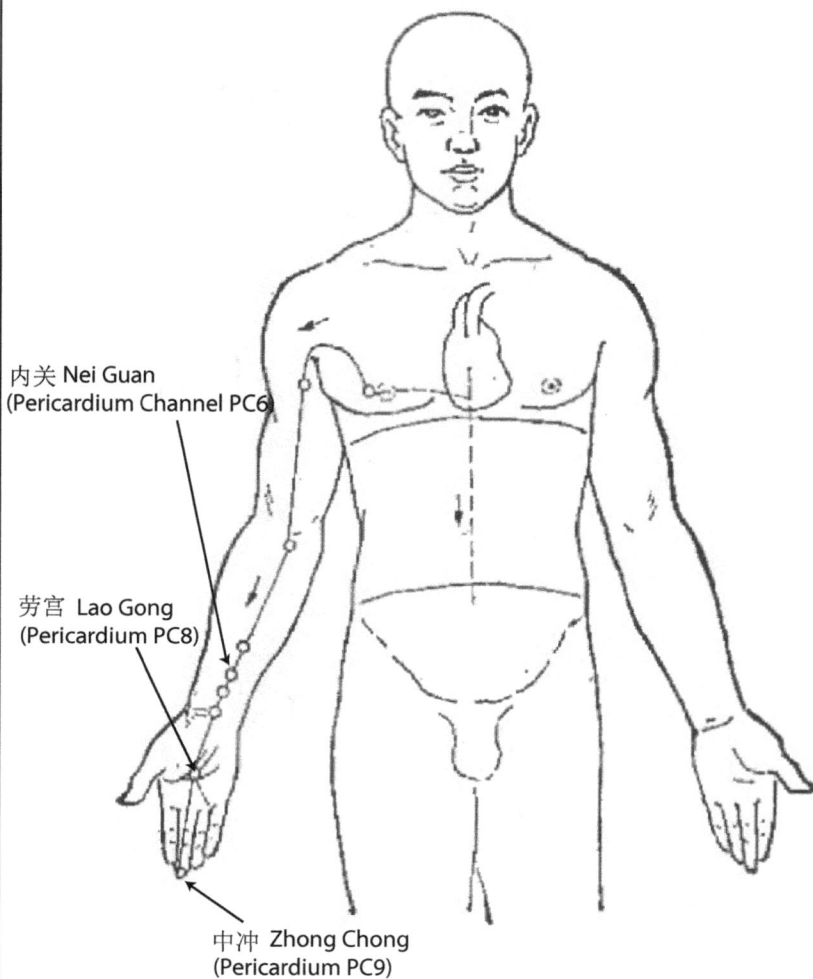

内关 Nei Guan
(Pericardium Channel PC6)

劳宫 Lao Gong
(Pericardium PC8)

中冲 Zhong Chong
(Pericardium PC9)

No 11. The Pericardium Meridian (Yin) originates next to the nipple and flows down the centre of the inside of the arm, finishing at the middle finger.

# 三焦经 Triple warmer Meridian

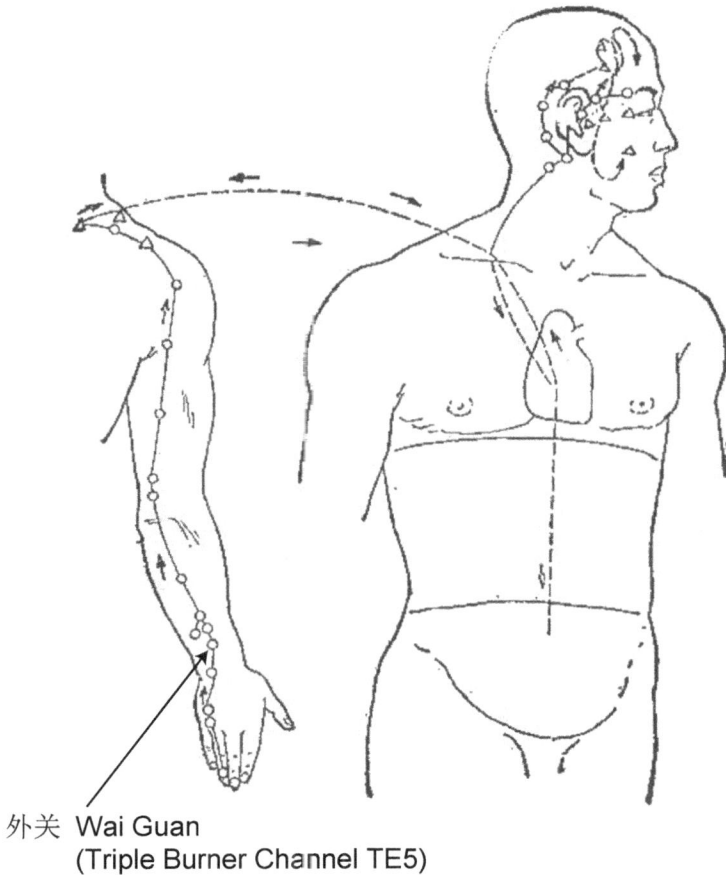

外关 Wai Guan
(Triple Burner Channel TE5)

No 12. The Triple Burner Meridian (Yang) starts at the tip of the ring finger, rises up the outside of the arm, the back of the shoulder to the collarbone, up the outside of the neck, and behind the ear before it dips down to the cheek and ends under the eye. An internal branch descends into the chest, through the diaphragm to the abdomen

# 督脉 Du Channel

百会 Bai Hui
(Governing Vessel GV20)

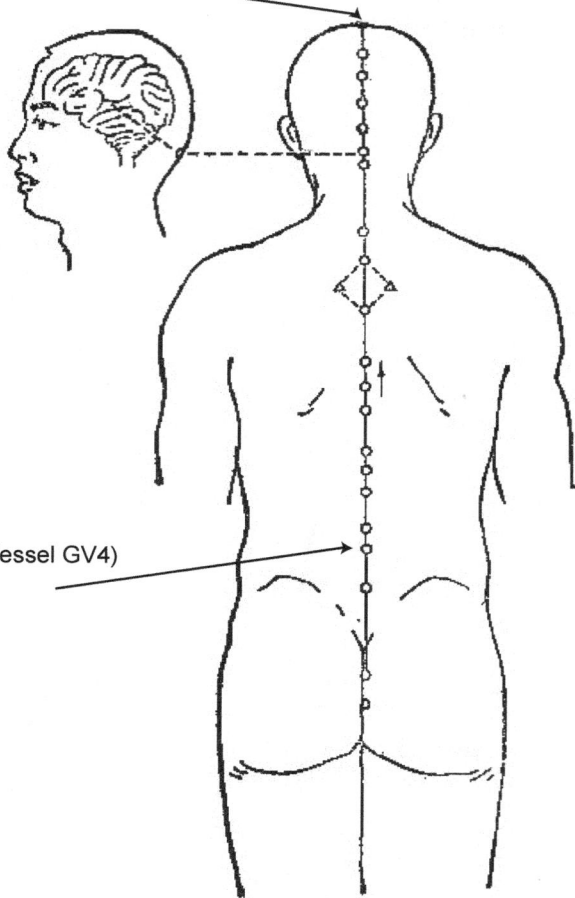

命门 Ming Men
(Governing Vessel GV4)

No 1. The Du Channel runs from the anus, up the spine and across the crown of the head to finish inside the upper lip.

# 任脉 Ren Channel

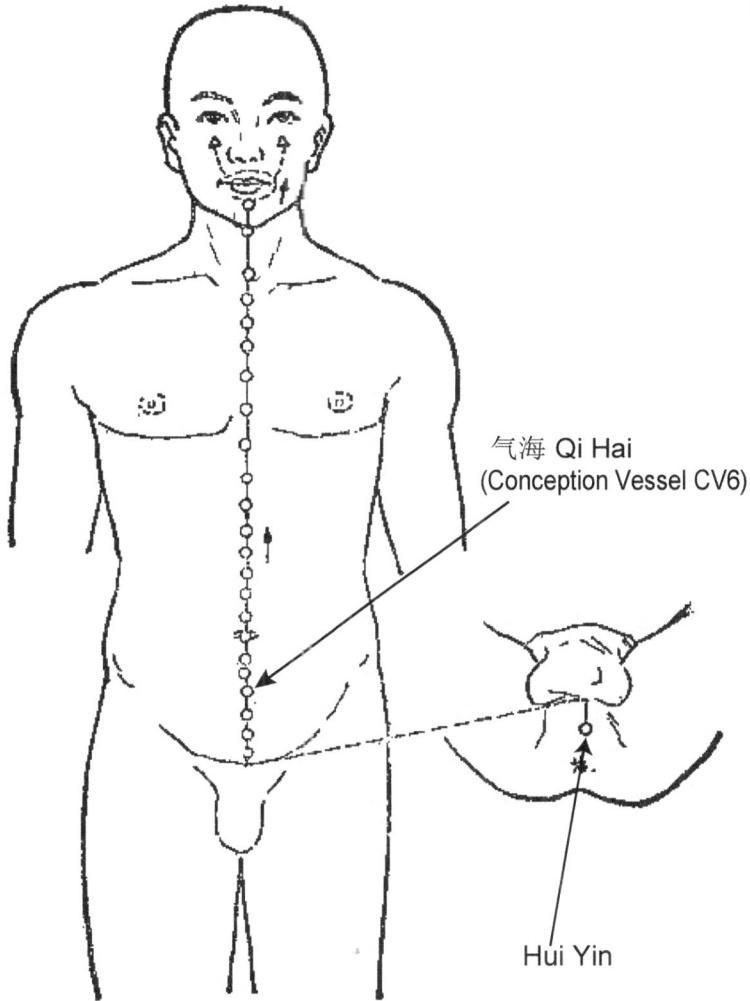

气海 Qi Hai
(Conception Vessel CV6)

Hui Yin

No 2. The Ren Channel originates in the uterus in females and in the lower abdomen in males and emerges at the Hui Yin in the perineum. It moves up the middle of the abdomen to the jaw, ending just below the lower lip.

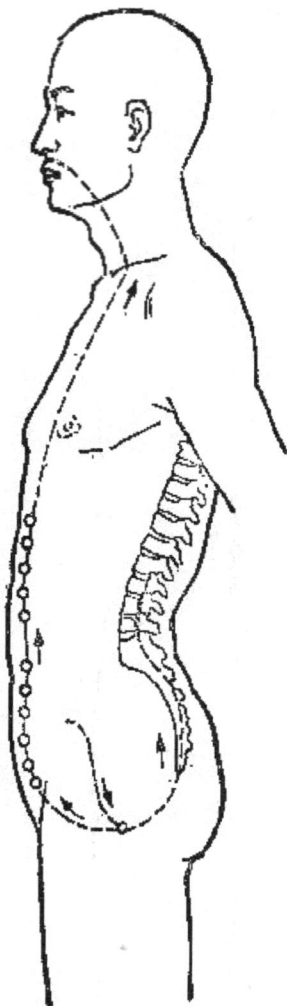

# 冲 脉 Chong Channel

No 3. The Chong Channel originates from inside the body to the perineum then ascends through the spine, the channel braches out along both sides of the abdomen up to the throat and finishing around the lips.

# 带脉 Dai Channel

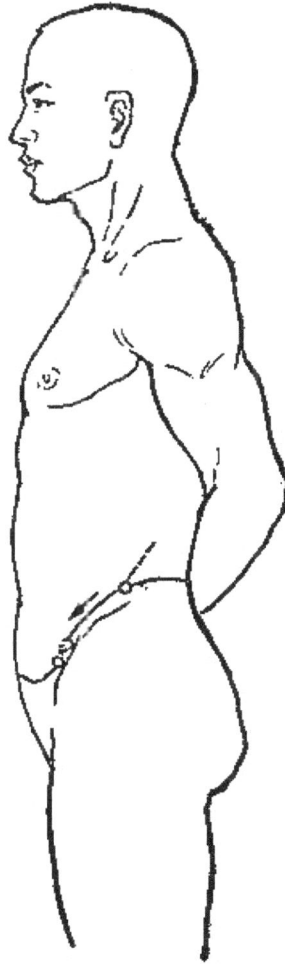

No 4. The Dai Channel (Girdle Vessel) runs around the waist like a belt.

# 阴跷脉 Yin Qiao Channel

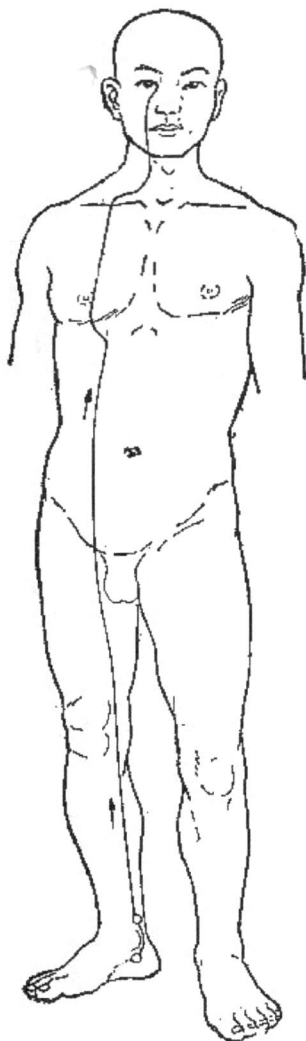

No 5. The Yin Qiao Channel travels along the inside of the heel and the leg, up the abdomen and the chest to the top of the collarbone. It passes along the throat, by the side of the mouth and nose, to the inner edge of the eye.

# 阳跷脉 Yang Qiao Channel

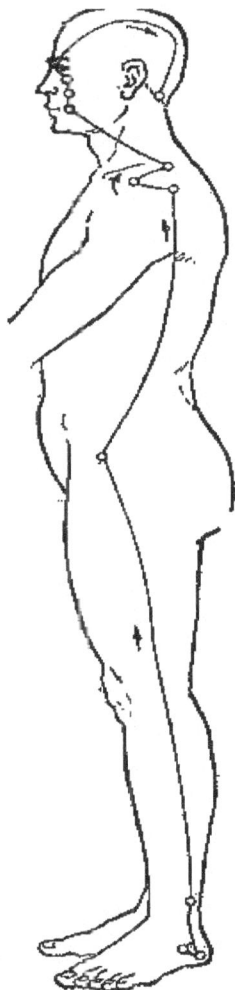

No 6. The Yang Qiao Channel, travels up the outside of the leg from the heel, to the thigh, the armpit, through the back of the shoulder and ascends the neck to the corner of the mouth, then passing over the head to finish at the nape of the neck.

# 阴维脉 Yin Wei Channel

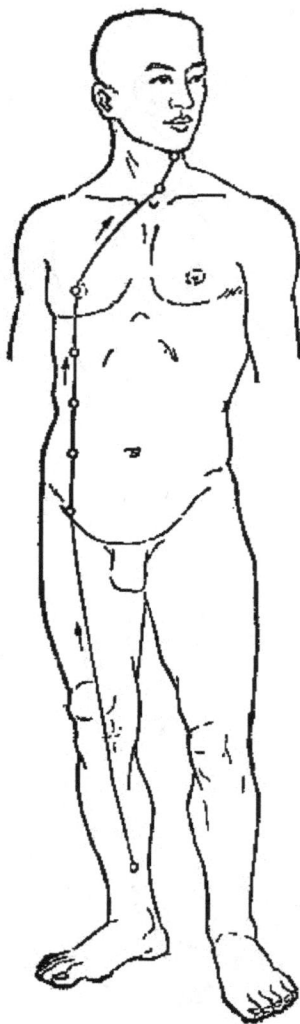

No 7. The Yin Wei Channel originates at the front of the leg, travels through the hip, over the chest and ends in the neck on the opposite side.

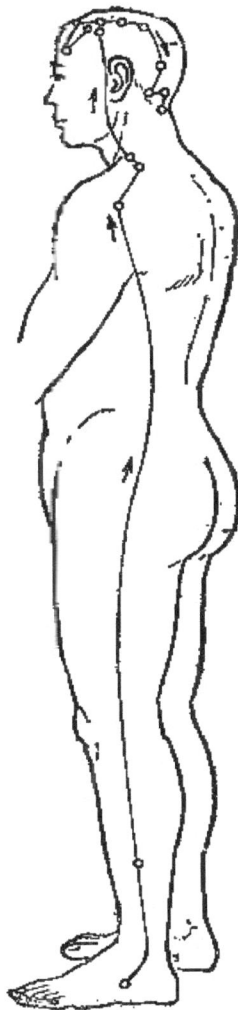

No 8. The Yang Wei Channel originates on the outside of the heel, moving up the outside of the leg to the hip, armpit, shoulder and neck. It then moves upwards to the cheeks and forehead then turns backwards to the back of the neck.

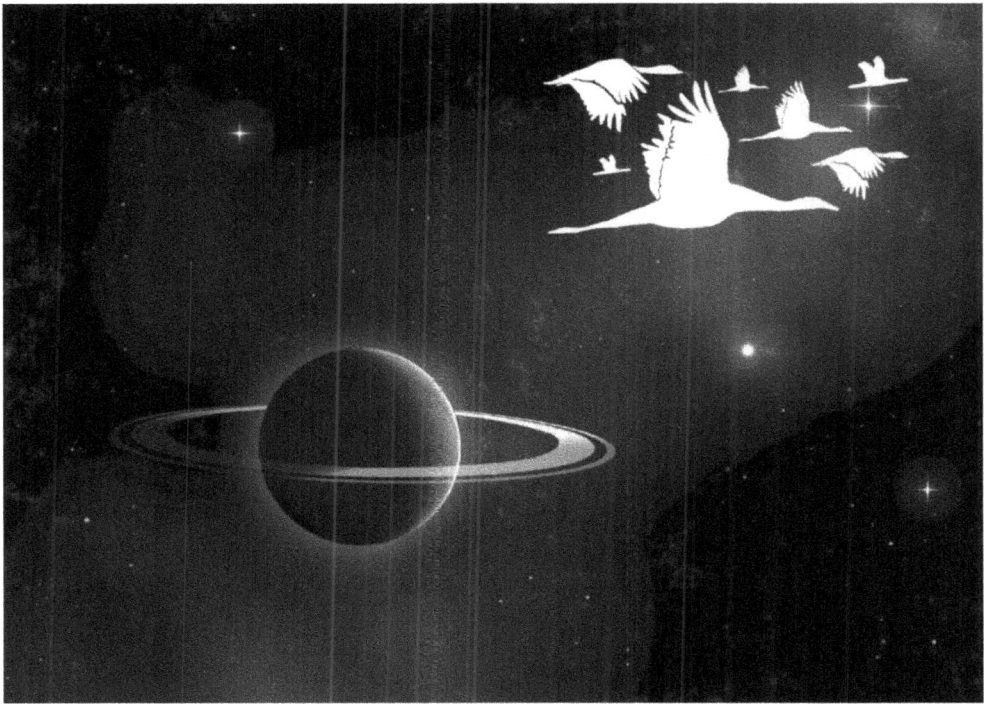

# Chapter 9
# INSPIRING STORIES

Da Yan - Wild Goose Qigong

The 2nd 64 movements

'I have been practising Qigong for sixteen years now and teaching it for five years. I practise nearly every day and feel restless if I don't.

'Sixteen years ago I was diagnosed with osteoporosis and shortly after that with osteoarthritis. I decided not to take any medication which had possible serious side effects and chose instead to try to heal myself with Qigong and the use of mineral and vitamin supplements. I have also had acupuncture treatments, often use acupressure on myself, have practised the heavenly orbit meditation regularly and have used Chinese herbs and ointments.

'When I saw Simon demonstrating the first Da Yan form a few years ago, I knew that I had to learn it. It felt like the right thing for me to do and so I let go of the other Qigong forms I had been practising for over ten years.

'I loved working under Master Chen in China for he seemed so strong and happy despite his advanced age. He was encouraging at all times but always made sure he corrected imprecise movements and mistakes. I felt my Da Yan got so much stronger from understanding his explanations on Qi flow and focus and I always felt an incredibly strong field of energy when he was working with us. I did not experience any of my crippling migraines despite the high heat and humidity and felt happy and balanced while I was there.

'Qigong is for me the cultivation of internal energy through movement, breathing, meditation and study. It nurtures the health of our whole being in which circulates the earth and heavenly Qi. It allows us to feel and be part of the universal energy which is in us and everywhere around us. It makes me feel complete and often fills me with inner peace and happiness.

'I feel it's keeping my osteoporosis at bay and helps me remain strong and flexible. My headaches and migraines have become less frequent and I rarely use painkillers nowadays. It has made me a much more balanced person both mentally and emotionally.

'I guess I have learnt to trust myself more, to feel more confident about my actions and intuitions. I have also learned that helping people feel happier through teaching and practice is one of my most important achievements, besides being a parent.

'Simon's greatest gift is his ability to make complex concepts so accessible to all people. His teaching is so clear yet so simple and profound that everybody feels included and encouraged to advance further. As a Qigong teacher this is what I hope to achieve in the future.'

**Sylvia, Tasmania**

'I have been practising Qigong for about thirty years and have always been more interested in the internal, rather than the external form. Qigong is a part of my life. I practise it every day and also attend class three times a week.

'I started Tai Chi classes when I was working full time and completing a master's degree. I felt pretty overloaded at the time. I found that Tai Chi helped me relax and made me more able to cope with my work and study load.

'When I attended my first class I was hooked. I started with the external form and somewhere on my journey I discovered the internal form. Learning, practising and teaching Qigong is now an integral part of my life. I just love the sense of peace and harmony that I am left with after I practise.
'Words can't explain how privileged I felt to be able to learn Da Yan Wild Goose from the 28th Generation lineage Grand Master. I honour and respect Master Chen as my lineage Grand Master. He is a wonderful, generous man who has a wealth of knowledge that he is more than happy to share. The icing on the cake is Master Chen's wonderful wife who also contributes to the teaching. Madam Chen is a kind, caring lady who I look forward to catching up with each time I visit Wuhan in China.

'I now take time to 'smell the roses'. I feel healthier. I am now more appreciative of life and my life has better balance. I am now more able to 'let go'. Where the mind goes the Qi follows. Anyone can practise Qigong.'

**Amber, New South Wales**


'I have been practising Qigong for more than ten years, and prior to that ten years of Tai Chi Chuan. I love my daily practice and at least five days each week I do a morning practice. I found a deeper connection with Qi when I started classes with Simon in Sydney in 2007. Since then I have been teaching Qigong on the Central Coast of NSW.

'My first trip with Simon to China included visiting Wuhan, and I was privileged to be one of twenty Westerners to learn Da Yan Wild Goose with Master Chen. This experience has profoundly influenced my life and teaching ever since.

'Grand Master Chen is an inspirational teacher and passionate about Da Yan Wild Goose. He is also patient and generous with his time. I loved his style; as we practised he would sit quietly, seemingly not watching, then he would stand and surprise us by knowing each person's weaker points, patiently showing us the movements, and then encouraging and praising us when we got it right. I have trained with him on three trips to China and loved every minute of the intensive training. Personally, it is a wonderful feeling knowing that at the end of the weeks' training with Simon and Master Chen, I had achieved some mastery of the form.

'I was so inspired by Grand Master Chen and the practice of Da Yan Wild Goose that I applied for and was accepted as a lineage student of the Master. I had my initiation with two others in 2013. My goal now is to teach as many people as I can, staying true to the lineage and form.
'Qigong is a powerful Chinese remedial exercise and is a comprehensive approach to health and wellbeing. When practised regularly the benefits are cumulative. They can be subtle yet provide a feeling of balance in the mind and body, plus a deep contentment.

'I feel a deep connection to Qi when practising, especially the Da Yan Wild Goose. I encourage my students to recognise the movement of energy in their bodies and to feel the Qi. When they do it is wonderful to see the smiles on their faces.

'Qigong allows me to be healthier, more disciplined with my practice and diet. When my mind is clear, I feel calm, less stressed, my energy levels are enhanced and I feel a vitality that I can only put down to my Qigong practice.

'Qigong has taught me to be more aware of how and what I feel, to listen to my body and to be kinder to myself. My Qigong practice has also given me the confidence to teach with diligence, and to inspire my students. Each day is a wonderful experience; life is good.
'Training with a Master like Simon Blow or Grand Master Chen is a must for any student of Qigong. It you get the opportunity, do it. You will have an experience you will never forget.'
**Cherel, New South Wales**


'I have been practising for one year, and I practise every day. My father started first and through him I became interested. It has helped my chronic gastritis.

'Qigong helps promote the circulation within the body and also connects the human body with its outer environment.

'Practising Qigong makes me feel warm, relaxed, light and emotionally positive. I believe it has also relieved pain from my neck and back. It is worth learning and practising persistently.'
**Ai, China**

'I have been practising the Chinese healing arts for about twelve years and I practise on average seven times per week. Qigong was part of the Tai Chi classes that I attended, and then I became more interested in the health benefits of Qigong. I had also been studying yoga and meditation for many years beforehand. I found Qigong especially beneficial in the grieving process after my youngest son died.

'As soon as I started Da Yan Wild Goose Qigong I felt connected to the form and the overall health benefit as I progressed through the 1st 64 movements and then the 2nd 64 movements.

'Learning with Grand Master Chen is a very special experience. His knowledge and understanding of Qigong is immeasurable. One gets the feeling of being in the presence of a true master of the form, yet he shows great patience and humility in the way he teaches. He also has a great sense of humour.

'Qigong is the study and cultivation of Qi or life energy in the body. It makes me feel energised yet relaxed. It certainly has a calming effect and I can deal with the ups and downs of modern life much better. I tend to not let the small things in life worry me and I live in the moment. Also it makes me feel stronger physically.

'I thank Master Simon Blow for his enthusiasm and commitment in his teaching. I enjoy the trips to China; they are a good mix of study and fun. Simon makes learning Qigong easy. He inspired me to become a 29th Generation student of Grand Master Chen and he made me realise that I could teach.'
**George, New South Wales**


'I have been practising Qigong for more than ten years and I practice three to six times a week. I had cancer treatment in 2002 and I wanted to maximise my health, both physically and mentally. I also think the meditation aspects of Qigong are part of a spiritual practice. Some other Chinese healing arts I have used include acupuncture, massage and herbal medicine.

'I was very drawn to the Da Yan Wild Goose because of its high energy. It was a natural development from the other Qigong forms that I had been working on. I enjoyed the focus and intensity of the work with Master Chen in China. It was both demanding and rewarding. I also appreciated the energy of working with other dedicated practitioners.

'Qigong is a meditative, grounding practice, coming out of both Daoist philosophy and Traditional Chinese Medicine. Qigong exercises the body, calms the mind and helps to connect mind, body and spirit.

'Qigong makes me feel calm, focused, happy and healthy. I have experienced improved health, both physically and mentally. I also experience an enjoyable connection with other people who value Qigong.

'I have learned that regular practice and a little self discipline is very helpful in building a healthy life. I think the discipline of learning the Da Yan Wild Goose Qigong has been beneficial for my memory, as it is a complex practice.'
**Jann, New South Wales**


'Qigong is my passion and has become my way of life.

'I have been a Qigong practitioner following a cancer diagnosis in 2008 and have been gradually building and expanding my theoretical and practical skills through attending workshops and retreats, including a tour to China.

'My philosophy and approach to daily living is using an integrated Traditional Chinese Medicine (TCM) model incorporating acupuncture, Chinese herbs, Tui Na and Qigong. The benefits accruing to me have included a revitalised spiritual awareness, reading and growing from studying Daoism and being overwhelmed by the transformative nature of my inner being, including a quiet stillness and an enjoyment of my natural surroundings.

'More than anything I have huge enthusiasm for wanting to share my knowledge with others and allow them to enjoy the healing that I have experienced.

'I have gained body strength, particularly in my legs and feet because I previously had difficulty standing for any length of time. My arthritic pain has reduced substantially, my blood pressure is controlled and my TCM practitioner has commented that there is less stagnation and a better flow of Qi through my meridians as a result of my regular Qigong practice. This means that there is less opportunity for blockages and illness to occur. I find myself smiling more and people commenting on this. My inner self seems to be shining through, something which I credit to daily Qigong practice.

'I have been involved with the Wild Goose since early 2013 and have found it an enjoyable challenge. The physical demands are quite energetic and the mental stamina required in learning the movements is rigorous. My journey is just beginning and I find my learning is greatly aided by the Master and more senior students. There is a genuine camaraderie amongst my fellow practitioners with all of us intent on mastering this form.
'Qigong consciousness transforms my inner being to infinity.'
**Sandi, New South Wales**

'I have been practising Qigong for about ten years and on average, I practise three times a week.

'I have studied acupuncture and Traditional Chinese Medicine and I understand and believe practising Qigong is good for a healthy body and mind. After reading an acupuncture medicine magazine it confirmed my decision to learn Qigong. It combines graceful movements and the stimulation of Qi flow in the body to improve health in a person.

'Learning from Master Chen gave me a deep understanding of what Da Yan Qigong means. I enjoyed his calmness, dedication and patience in passing on his knowledge and wisdom to students. It encouraged me to learn and understand more about Da Yan Qigong.

'To me Qigong is meditation in movement. The flow of Qi from the universe through my body and back to Mother Earth makes a full cycle like Yin and Yang in balance. The mind is still, the breathing natural and the movements slow and graceful. Therefore it joins the body, mind and spirit.

'It makes me feel calm, at peace, relaxed and my energy is replenished. There is a feeling of joy within. The philosophy and wisdom of Qigong helps me see what is happening around me in a different light.

'Experiencing the benefits of practicing Da Yan Qigong makes me want to share this 'good thing' with others. Not just the beautiful and precious movements but also the flow of Qi within the body. I want to pass on its philosophy to others too. This is the whole package of Qigong.

'I honour Simon as a true Master. I thank him from the bottom of my heart for his great work in promoting Qigong. Because of his belief in sharing the goodness and benefits of practising Qigong, many of us have the opportunity to go to China to learn Qigong. On behalf of many of your students, I thank you once again.'

**Janita, New South Wales**

# CDs – by Simon Blow

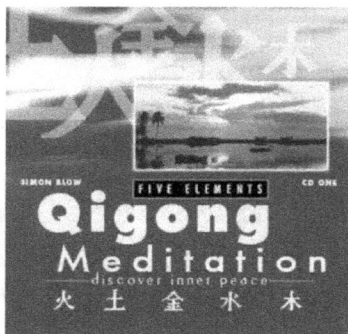

## CD1: Five Elements Qigong Meditation

This CD is the perfect introduction to Qigong meditation (Neigong). **Track one** features a 30-minute heart-felt guided meditation to help bring love and light from the universe into your body. It harmonises the Five Elements – Fire, Earth, Metal, Water and Wood – with the corresponding organs of the body, respectively the heart, spleen, lungs, kidney and liver. This is one of the foundations of Chinese Qigong. Let Qigong Master Simon Blow help harmonise the elements of the universe with the energy of your body by using colour and positive images. **Track two** provides 30 minutes of relaxing music by inspiring composer Dale Nougher.

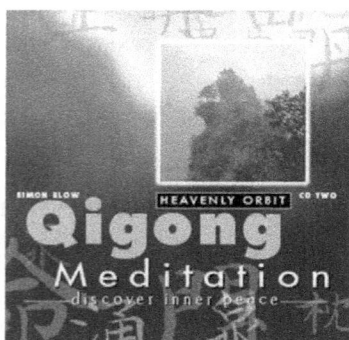

## CD2: Heavenly Orbit Qigong Meditation

This CD is intended for the intermediate student. **Track one** takes you through a 30-minute guided meditation using your awareness to stimulate the energy centres around the body and open all the meridians. The circulation of Qi (Chi) around the Heavenly Orbit is one of the foundations of Chinese Qigong. The energy rising up the back 'Du' channel harmonises with the energy descending down the front 'Ren' channel, helping balance the energy of the body. Master Simon Blow guides you to open the energy centres of your own body to create harmony with the universe. **Track two** provides 30 minutes of relaxing music by Dale Nougher.

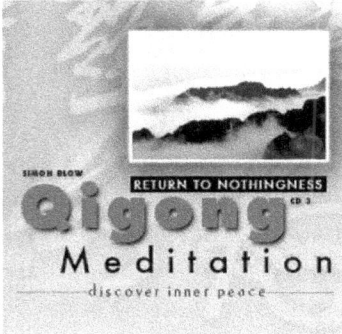

## CD3: Return to Nothingness Qigong Meditation

This CD is intended for the advanced student and those wanting a healing night-practice. One of the aims of Qigong is to allow our internal energy (Qi) to harmonise with the external energy (Qi) allowing our consciousness to merge with the universe. When we enter into a deep sleep or meditation all the meridians start to open and much healing can take place. In this 20-minute guided meditation Simon Blow assists you in guiding your energy through your body and harmonising with the energy of the universe. Track two provides 30 minutes of healing music by Dale Nougher.

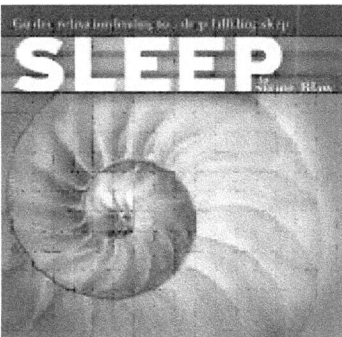

## Sleep

Sleep is necessary to maintain life, alongside breathing, eating, drinking, and exercising of the mind and body. Without a good six to eight hours of sleep each night it can be hard to live a quality, balanced, fulfilling life. When we sleep it's a time to rest and rejuvenate the mind and body and to release the physical, mental and emotional stress that has built up during the day. This also helps uplift us spiritually.

It's a time to rest; it's time for a good night's sleep. Let Simon Blow's soothing voice, along with Dale Nougher's beautiful piano music and the natural sounds of the ocean, help guide you to release the tension of the day and enable you to enter a deep, fulfilling sleep.

# Book/DVD sets – by Simon Blow

*"About 18 months ago I started to practise Qigong as I knew that it would improve my health. I needed to do it regularly, ideally every day, but being in a rural area presented logistical problems. I discovered Simon's DVD and commenced daily practice. The great advantage for me was that I didn't have to travel to classes and could do them whenever I felt like it. Since that time I have noticed great improvement in my overall wellbeing. It has helped me to reinvent my clinical practice as a holistic massage practitioner. A number of my clients now have Simon's DVD and I feel this is helping them to both improve their health and well being, and to empower themselves."* **Robin Godson-King (Holistic Massage Practitioner)**

**(Each set contains a DVD plus a book that provides diagrams and instructions for the movements contained on the DVD. The book also includes interesting reading about the practice of Qigong as well as inspirational stories.)**

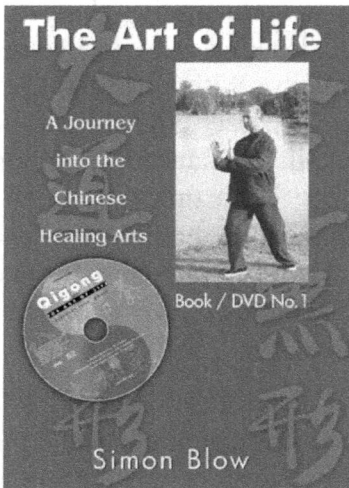

## The Art of Life

'The Art of Life' presents the Qigong styles that were taught to me in Australia: the Taiji Qigong Shibashi, which I learned as an instructor with the Australian Academy of Tai Chi from 1990 to 1995; and the Ba Duan Jin standing form, commonly known as the Eight Pieces of Brocade, taught to me in 1996 by Sifu John Dolic in Sydney.

This is the perfect introduction to this ancient art and is suitable for new and continuing students of all ages. The book follows the DVD and contains three sections: **1. Warm up** – gentle movements loosen all the major joints of the body, lubricating the tendons and helping increase blood and energy circulation. It is beneficial for most arthritic conditions; **2. Ba Duan Jin or Eight Pieces of Brocade** – this is the best known and most widely practised form of Qigong throughout the world, also known as Daoist Yoga. The movements stretch all the major muscles, massage organs and open the meridians of the body; **3. Taiji Qigong Shibashi** – this popular practice is made up of eighteen flowing movements. The gentle movements harmonise the mind, body and breath. Total running time: 55 minutes.

*"Tai Chi Qigong is a gentle way of exercising the whole body and provides long-term benefits. I recommend it to my patients as an effective way of improving muscle tone and joint mobility. Those who practise regularly have fewer problems with their muscles and joints and often report an increased sense of health and wellbeing. This is an excellent video with clear and simple instruction."*

**Roman Maslak. B.A. (Hons), D.O. Osteopath**

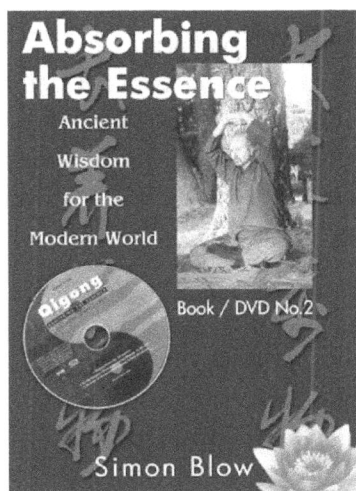

## Absorbing the Essence

'Absorbing the Essence' comprises the Qigong cultivation techniques that were taught to me by Grand Master Zhong Yunlong in 1999 and 2000 at Wudangshan or Wudang Mountain. Wudang is one of the sacred Daoist Mountains of China and is renowned for the development of Taiji.

This DVD and book is for the intermediate student and for people with experience in meditation. It contains three sections: **1. Warm up** – the same as in The Art of Life DVD; **2. Wudang Longevity Qigong** – this sequence of gentle, flowing movements stimulates the Heavenly Orbit, absorbing the primordial energy from the environment and letting the negativity dissolve into the distance; **3. Sitting Ba Duan Jin** – this 30-minute sequence includes eight sections with exercises to stimulate different organs and meridians of the body. It is practised in a seated position on a chair or cushion – ideal for people who have discomfort whilst standing. These practices originated from the famous Purple Cloud Monastery at the sacred Wudang Mountain in China. Total running time: 60 minutes.

*"Simon Blow of Australia has twice travelled (1999, 2000) to Mt Wudang Shan Daoist Wushu College to learn Taiji Hunyuan Zhuang (Longevity) Qigong and Badajin Nurturing Life Qigong and through his study has absorbed the essence of these teachings. Therefore, I specially grant Simon the authority to teach these, spreading the knowledge of these Qigong methods he has learnt at Mt Wudang to contribute to the wellbeing of the human race. May the Meritorious Deeds Be Infinite."*

**Grand Master Zhong Yunlong, Daoist Priest and Director,**
**Mt Wudang Shan Taoist Wushu College, China, September 24, 2000.**

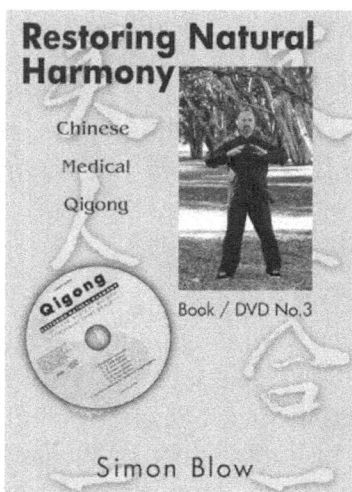

## Restoring Natural Harmony

This DVD and book is for the advanced student or for the person wanting to learn specific Traditional Chinese Medicine self-healing exercises. Each section works on a different organ meridian system of the body – Spleen, Lungs, Kidney, Liver and Heart – which relate to the Five Elements – Earth, Metal, Water, Wood and Fire. Guigen Qigong originated from Dr Xu Hongtao, a Qigong Specialist Doctor from the Xiyuan Hospital in Beijing. These internal exercises help regulate the meridian system bringing harmony to mind, body and spirit. Total running time: 75 minutes.

*"Simon Blow first visited our hospital in 2002. I was impressed with his knowledge and commitment to Qigong. He returned in 2004 to study Chinese Medical Qigong. Simon is a gifted teacher: he has the rare ability to inspire others and impart to them the healing benefits of Qigong."*
**Dr Xu Hongtao, Qigong and Tuina Department, Xiyuan Hospital Beijing, China.**

*"This DVD – the third by the impressively qualified Sydney-based Simon Blow – serves two purposes. Firstly, it is so attractively produced that the curious would surely be induced to investigate further. Secondly, for those already practising, it provides a mnemonic device much more useful than a series of still pictures."* **Review by Adyar Bookshop, Sydney 2005.**

**These are not medical devices and should not be used to replace any existing medical treatment. Always consult with your health provider if uncertain.**

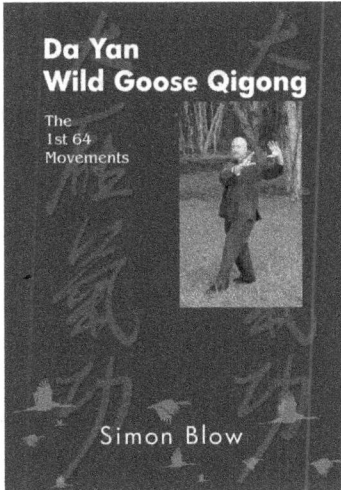

# Da Yan Wild Goose Qigong
## The first 64 movements

'Da Yan' translates to 'great bird' and is an ancient cultivation practice originating from the Jin Dynasty about 1700 years ago. Daoist Masters from the sacred Kunlun Mountains, in the Northern Himalayan area in south-west China, would observe the migrating geese which descended in this area each year. They would mimic the movements of these great birds and started to developed the Da Yan Wild Goose Qigong system.

Its healing and spiritual legacy was passed down through many generations; however Dayan Qigong was withheld from the general public until 1978. Then 27th lineage holder Grand Master Yang Mei Jung (1895-2002) decided to teach this ancient Qigong practice and share its healing benefits to improve the quality of life of all people.

The 1st 64 movement set deals primary with the 'post-natal body' relating to the energy that one gathers after birth. The movements representing the flight of wild geese are slow, graceful movements and strong, quick movements designed to release stale Qi and to gather fresh Qi, helping to restore balance and stimulate the entire energy system of the body.

*'I've benefitted in many ways from Qigong. In physical terms, I'm stronger, have better balance and coordination and my muscles and joints are moving freely. I can recognise symptoms of anxiety and use my practice to slow things down in my mind and body when it all gets too hectic. Qigong is also a wonderful aid to recovery from illness and surgery.'* **Joy**

*'I am finding it easier to focus on present tasks, listen more and have a satisfying spiritual connection throughout the day.'* **Wendy**

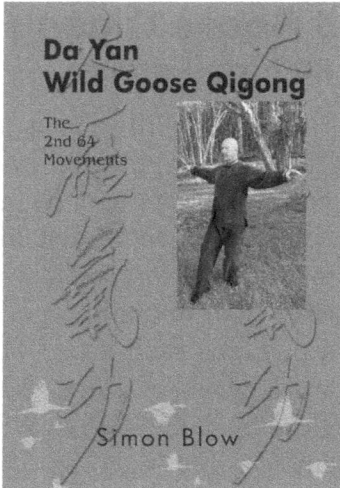

# Da Yan Wild Goose Qigong
## The second 64 movements

From ancient times, Qigong was an important component of the Chinese medical health system, and developed to help improve people's quality of life. The art of Qigong consists primarily of meditation, relaxation, physical movement, mind-body integration and breathing exercises. When the mind and body come into a state of balance, stress is reduced and there is an increase in health and longevity.

The 2nd 64 movement set of Da Yan Wild Goose Qigong deals primarily with the 'pre-natal body', which refers to the energy we gather from the universe and from our ancestors before birth. Having dredged the channels in the 1st 64 movement set, the 2nd 64 movement set is designed to clear the channels to absorb fresh Qi, expel stale Qi and to restore organ balance. The twisting, stretching, bending and pressing movements produce stronger Qi fields and intensify the circulation through the energy channels. In the 2nd 64 movement set, the Goose embarks on a great journey and flies out from this world to the edge of the Milky Way to pick herbs or gather pre-natal Qi from the core of the universe. It then flies back to this world to share this healing energy with humanity.

*'Simon's greatest gift is his ability to make complex concepts so accessible to all people. His teaching is so clear yet so simple and profound that everybody feels included and encouraged to advance further. As a Qigong teacher this is what I hope to achieve in the future.'* **Sylvia**

*'Qigong has taught me to be more aware of how and what I feel; to listen to my body and to be kinder to myself. My Qigong practice has also given me the confidence to teach with diligence, and to inspire my students. Each day is a wonderful experience; life is good.'* **Cherel**

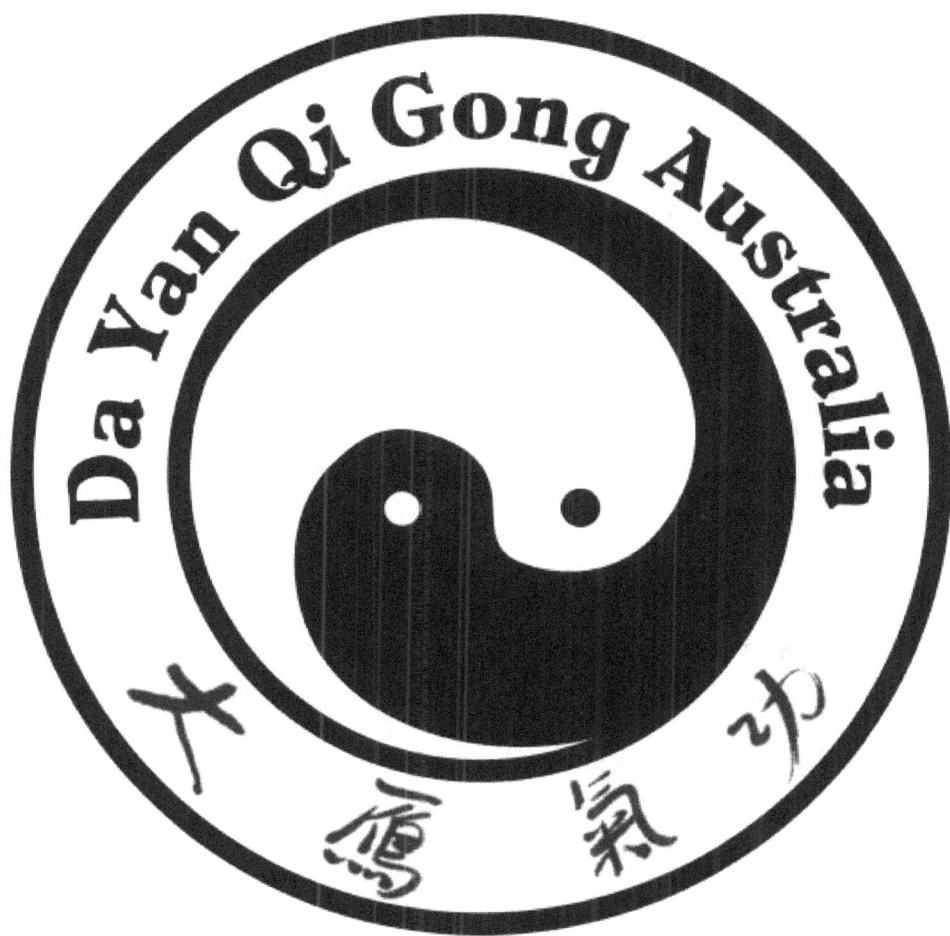

# ☯ Simon Blow Qigong 信思

## — for better health and inner peace —

## To order products or for more information on:

- Regular classes in Sydney for new and continuing students
- Workshops or if you would be interested in helping organise a workshop in your local area
- Residential Qigong and Meditation retreats
- China Qigong Study Tours for students and advanced training
- Talks, corporate classes, training and presentations
- Wholesale enquiries

## Please contact:

**Simon Blow**
PO Box 446
Summer Hill, NSW 2130
Sydney Australia

Ph: +61 (0)2 9559 8153

Web: **www.simonblowqigong.com**

**CDs and Book/DVDs can be ordered online and shipped nationally and internationally.**

# Bibliography

Yang Meijun, *Wild Goose Qigong*. China: China Science and Technology Press. 1991

Liu TJ, Chen KW et al. (eds) *Chinese Medical Qigong*. London: Singing Dragon. 2010.

Ni Hua-Ching. *Esoteric Tao Teh Ching*. California: Seven Star Communications Group, Inc., 1992.

Ni Hua-Ching. *The Gentle Path of Spiritual Progress*. California: Shrine of the Eternal Breath of Tao, 1987

Ellis, Wiseman, Boss. *Grasping the Wind*. Massachusetts: Paradigm Publications , 1989

Yang, Jwing-Ming. *The Root of Chinese Qigong*, Massachusetts: YMAA Publication Centre, 1997.
Blow Simon. *The Art of Life*. Sydney: Genuine Wisdom Centre, 2010
Blow Simon. *Absorbing the Essence*. Sydney: Genuine Wisdom Centre, 2010
Blow Simon. *Restoring Natural Harmony*. Sydney: Genuine Wisdom Centre, 2010
Basic *Theory of Traditional Chinese Medicine*. China: Publishing House of Shanghai University of Traditional Chinese Medicine, 2002.

Liu, Qingshan. *Chinese Fitness*. Massachusetts: YMAA Publication Centre, 1997.

Magpie Goose People story Copyright © George Milpurrurru

## Websites

www.wikipedia.org
www.esotericastrologer.org
www.eng.taoism.org.hk
www.dierinbeeld.nl/animal_files/birds/goose/
www.egreenway.com/taichichuan/goose.htm
www.chinaonlinemuseum.com

Meridian charts originally sourced from Basic Theory of Traditional Chinese Medicine. China: Publishing House of Shanghai University of Traditional Chinese Medicine. 1988

Meridian Acupoints originally sourced
www.cgicm.ca/cn
www.en.tcm-china
www.acupuncture.com
www.thedaoofdragonball.com
www.compassionatedragon.com
www.ttpacupuncture.com
www.shen-nong.com
www.buzzle.com